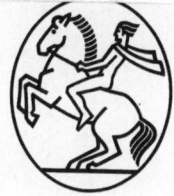

Lesions of the Cerebral Midline

9th Scientific Meeting of the European Society
for Paediatric Neurosurgery (ESPN),
October 10–13, 1984, Vienna

Edited by W. T. Koos
and G. Pendl

Acta Neurochirurgica
Supplementum 35

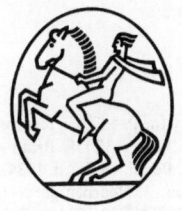

Springer-Verlag Wien New York

Dr. Wolfgang T. Koos, Professor of Neurosurgery
Dr. Gerhard Pendl, Associate Professor of Neurosurgery
Department of Neurosurgery, University of Vienna Medical School, Wien, Austria

With 128 Figures

Library of Congress Cataloging-in-Publication Data. European Society for Paediatric Neurosurgery. Scientific Meeting (9th: 1984: Vienna, Austria). Lesions of the cerebral midline. (Acta neurochirurgica. Supplementum, ISSN 0065-1419; 35.) 1. Brain—Tumors—Congresses. 2. Brain—Tumors—Surgery—Congresses. 3. Tumors in children—Surgery—Congresses. I. Koos, Wolfgang Th. II. Pendl, Gerhard, 1934-   . III. Title. IV. Series. [DNLM: 1. Brain Neoplasms—diagnosis—congresses. 2. Brain Neoplasms—in infancy & childhood—congresses. 3. Neurosurgery—in infancy & childhood—congresses. W1 AC8661 no. 35/WL 358 E89 1984L]. RC280.B7E87 1984. 617'.481. 85-27607.

ISSN 0065-1419
ISBN-13:978-3-211-81883-1   e-ISBN-13:978-3-7091-8813-2
DOI: 10.1007/978-3-7091-8813-2

Preface

This supplement to "Acta Neurochirurgica" contains a selection of papers which were presented at the 9th Scientific Meeting of the European Society for Paediatric Neurosurgery on Space Occupying Lesions of the Cerebral Midline in Vienna, October 10–13, 1984. This meeting was arranged at the same location where the ESPN was founded exactly seventeen years ago. Although the presentations in this meeting dealt with numerous important problems encountered in paediatric neurosurgery, the main emphasis was on that special problem which exemplifies the extraordinary advances in paediatric neurosurgery and its related fields. Therefore the main topic of this scientific meeting was dedicated to the subject of "Space Occupying Lesions of the Cerebral Midline". Recent diagnostic procedures, such as computerized axial tomography and magnetic resonance imaging, now enable the neurosurgeon preoperatively, to obtain precise data on the location, and in many cases also on the nature of a lesion deep within the brain. Fundamental new knowledge in neuroanatomy and neurotopography has now transformed previous high-risk procedures into routine ones for the neurosurgeon, and an abundance of new surgical techniques has improved the success rate in the treatment of many patients. The scientific meetings of the ESPN have proved to be a successful forum for the exchange of experiences, opinions and even critical discussions. The present selection of papers will undoubtedly support this endeavour.

Wolfgang T. Koos
Gerhard Pendl

Contents

Contents

Acta Neurochirurgica, Suppl. 35, 1–5 (1985)

A. Statistics

Statistics of Intracranial Midline Tumors in Children

W. T. Koos and **A. Horaczek**

Department of Neurosurgery, University of Vienna Medical School, Wien, Austria

Summary

Of the 1,280 pediatric brain tumors seen at the Department of Neurosurgery, University of Vienna, until December 1984 57% involved the midline. Midline tumors were supratentorial in 40% of cases and infratentorial in 60%. The distribution of different tumor types in the various anatomical regions follows the known sites of predilection of brain tumors. Orienting diagrams show their rates in numerical terms, in various regions as well as their "clinical" malignancy.

Keywords: Pediatric brain tumors; midline tumors; tumor types; "clinical" malignancy.

The term "intracranial midline" stands for a considerable number of diagnostic and surgical problems associated with the complicated neuroanatomy and neurotopography of this region as well as the pathomorphology of the tumors encountered there.

The authors therefore, think it is appropriate to make some contribution to major problems in the diagnosis and treatment of midline tumors based on some fundamental statistical data, which were obtained from the patient population at the Department of Neurosurgery of the University of Vienna[8, 9, 10, 11, 12, 15].

Brain tumors were encountered in 1,280 children and juvenile patients at the Vienna Department of Neurosurgery until autumn 1984. Of these, 733 (57%) tumors were located in the intracranial midline (Table 1). 291 (40%) were situated above the tentorium, 442 (60%) were infratentorial (Table 2).

In terms of the topographic anatomy, the surgeon deals with the following regions and their anatomical structures: The supratentorial "midline" includes the sella turcica-optic chiasm region. Here, particularly the

Table 1. *Incidence of Intracranial Midline Tumors in the Series of Pediatric Brain Tumor Cases from the Department of Neurosurgery of the Vienna University*

NEUROSURGICAL UNIVERSITY CLINIC VIENNA 1984	
INTRACRANIAL TUMORS OF INFANTS AND CHILDREN	
TOTAL NUMBER OF CASES	1280
MIDLINE TUMORS	733 (57%)

Table 2. *Frequency of Midline Brain Tumors According to their Supra- and Infratentorial Location*

NEUROSURGICAL UNIVERSITY CLINIC VIENNA 1984		
INTRACRANIAL TUMORS OF INFANTS AND CHILDREN MIDLINE TUMORS		
	NO. OF CASES	%
SUPRATENTORIAL TUMORS	291	40
INFRATENTORIAL TUMORS	442	60
TOTAL	733	100

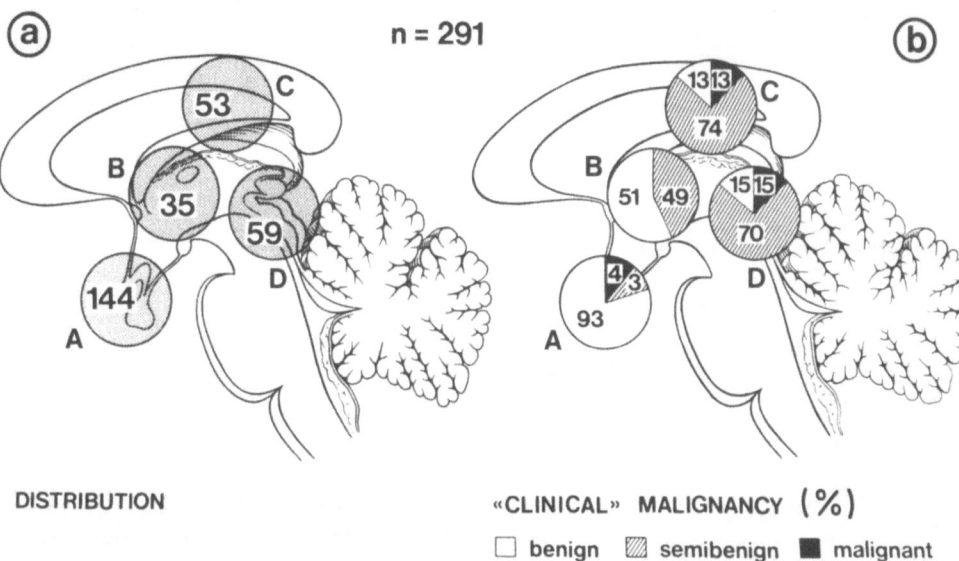

NEUROSURGICAL UNIVERSITY CLINIC VIENNA 1984

SUPRATENTORIAL MIDLINE TUMORS IN CHILDREN

PEDIATRIC BRAIN TUMOR COLLECTION   TOTAL: n = 1280 CASES

Fig. 1a, b. a Schematic drawing of the regional distribution of the tumors of the optic chiasm-sella turcica region (A), the third ventricle (B), the pineal and quadrigeminal plate region (D), and the paraventricular tumors which originate from the thalamus and the basal ganglia and extend into the ventricular lumen (C). b Distribution of supratentorial midline tumors according to their "clinical" malignancy

suprasellar infra- and retrochiasmal lesions growing towards the third ventricle present major surgical problems.

Other regions are the third ventricle[6, 9, 10, 11, 12, 21], where the surgeon deals both with tumors that primarily develop intraventricularly[2, 4, 6, 12, 16, 12], and blastomas with secondary growth into the ventricle from the wall and adjacent structures (paraventricular tumors)[9, 10, 12]. The tumors of the pineal and quadrigeminal plate region have always been of special interest to the surgeon[1, 3, 5, 7, 8, 9, 12, 17, 18]. Until recently, midbrain tumors were considered inoperable (Fig. 1).

Tumors of the infratentorial midline are fare more frequent and less complicated in terms of surgical technique, since they are easily accessible and there is little danger to harm vital anatomical structures when approaching them. These are the tumors of the cerebellar vermis, the fourth ventricle and, to a certain extent, tumors of the brainstem (Fig. 2).

Tables 3a and b present a survey of the tumor types encountered in the supra- and infratentorial midline. In these tables, the predilection of certain tumor types for certain areas of the brain is well seen, as suggested in previous publications[12, 13, 14, 15, 19, 20, 24, 27].

In evaluating the degree of malignancy of brain tumors, morphological characteristics alone will not give the clinician any practical useful indications as to the most appropriate therapeutic strategy to be followed as well as to the assessment of the patient's fate.

Thus, the morphologically determined malignancy has to be distinguished from the "clinical" malignancy, which is determined by the triad: intrinsic or genuine growth properties of the tumor - the site of the tumor— and the age of onset[11, 13, 18, 21, 22, 25].

It goes without saying that these two concepts may differ substantially from case to case. The differentiation of morphological and clinical malignancy proved of particular significance in the tumors of the central nervous system, where every histologically benign tumor may, in the long run, prove to be clinically malignant, i.e. constitute a danger to health and life of the patient[20, 24].

An evaluation of the "clinical" malignancy of the tumors encountered in the intracranial midline in the previously mentioned regions is shown in Tables 4, 5, 6, and 7, and in Figs. 1 and 2[12, 13, 14].

It is striking to note that supratentorial tumors are predominantly benign, and infratentorial neoplasms are largely malignant. It should be pointed out that evaluation of the biology or clinical malignancy of brain tumors dates back to the "premicrosurgical" era of the treatment of brain tumors[8, 10, 11, 18, 22]. Today, new neurosurgical techniques, and/or stereotactic interstitial tumor radiation, have improved the patient's prognosis, his survival time and quality of life.

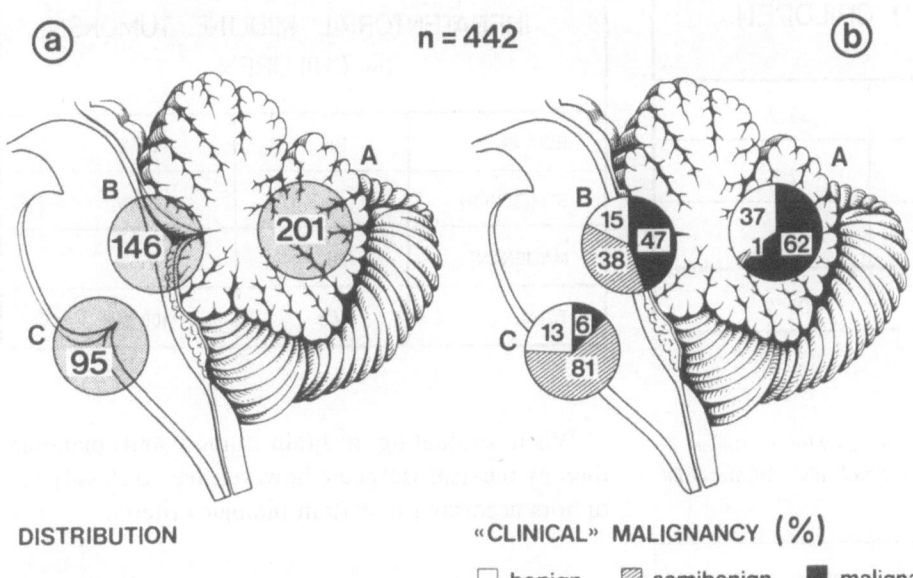

NEUROSURGICAL UNIVERSITY CLINIC VIENNA 1984

INFRATENTORIAL MIDLINE TUMORS IN CHILDREN

PEDIATRIC BRAIN TUMOR COLLECTION   TOTAL: n = 1280 CASES

n = 442

DISTRIBUTION

"CLINICAL" MALIGNANCY (%)

☐ benign   ▨ semibenign   ■ malignant

Fig. 2a, b. a Schematic drawing of the regional distribution of the midline tumors of the posterior cranial fossa, i.e. tumors of the cerebellar vermis (A), the fourth ventricle (B), and the brainstem (C). b Distribution of infratentorial midline brain tumors according to their "clinical" malignancy

Table 3a. *Incidence of Supratentorial Midline Brain Tumors in Children*

NEUROSURGICAL UNIVERSITY CLINIC VIENNA 1984	
INTRACRANIAL TUMORS OF INFANTS AND CHILDREN	
SUPRATENTORIAL MIDLINE TUMORS	
TYPE OF TUMOR	NO. OF CASES
CRANIOPHARYNGIOMAS	83
SPONGIOBLASTOMAS	42
ASTROCYTOMAS	39
PINEALOMAS	17
PITUITARY ADENOMAS	10
PINEOBLASTOMAS	9
EPENDYMOMAS	7
TERATOMAS	6
RETINOBLASTOMAS	5
GLIOBLASTOMAS	5
DERMOIDS/EPIDERMOIDS	5
GERMINOMAS	3
SARCOMAS	3
OLIGODENDROGLIOMAS	2
GRANULOMAS	2
OSTEOMAS	2
TUMORS OF LOCALIZED OSTEITIS FIBROSA	2
MENINGIOMAS	1
GANGLIOGLIOMAS	1
HEMANGIOBLASTOMAS	1
HAMARTOMAS	1
ANEURYSMS, SPACEOCCUPYING	4
SPACEOCCUPYING CYSTS	5
UNCLASSIFIED TUMORS	36
TOTAL	291

Table 3b. *Incidence of Infratentorial Midline Brain Tumors in Children*

NEUROSURGICAL UNIVERSITY CLINIC VIENNA 1984	
INTRACRANIAL TUMORS OF INFANTS AND CHILDREN	
INFRATENTORIAL MIDLINE TUMORS	
TYPE OF TUMOR	NO. OF CASES
MEDULLOBLASTOMAS	190
CEREBELLAR ASTROCYTOMAS	84
EPENDYMOMAS	47
ASTROCYTOMAS	46
SPONGIOBLASTOMAS	10
GLIOBLASTOMAS	6
SARCOMAS	4
CHOROID PLEXUS PAPILLOMAS	4
HEMANGIOBLASTOMAS	3
TUBERCULOMAS	1
DERMOIDS/EPIDERMOIDS	1
HAMARTOMAS	1
CHORDOMAS	1
SPACEOCCUPYING CYSTS	3
UNCLASSIFIED TUMORS	41
TOTAL	442

Table 4. *"Clinical" Malignancy of Midline Brain Tumors in Children*

NEUROSURGICAL UNIVERSITY CLINIC VIENNA 1984 MIDLINE TUMORS IN CHILDREN		
BENIGN	276	38 %
SEMIBENIGN	235	32 %
MALIGNANT	222	30 %
TOTAL	733	100 %

Table 7. *"Clinical" Malignancy of Infratentorial Midline Tumors*

NEUROSURGICAL UNIVERSITY CLINIC VIENNA 1984 INFRATENTORIAL MIDLINE TUMORS IN CHILDREN		
BENIGN	108	58 %
SEMIBENIGN	134	30 %
MALIGNANT	200	45 %
TOTAL	442	100 %

Table 5. *"Clinical" Malignancy of Intracranial Midline Tumors in Children According to Their Supratentorial and Infratentorial Location*

NEUROSURGICAL UNIVERSITY CLINIC VIENNA 1984 INTRACRANIAL TUMORS OF INFANTS AND CHILDREN MIDLINE TUMORS			
"CLINICAL" MALIGNANCY	SUPRATENTORIAL	INFRATENTORIAL	NO. OF CASES
BENIGN	168	108	276
SEMIBENIGN (SEMIMALIGNANT)	101	134	235
MALIGNANT	22	200	222
TOTAL	291	442	733

When evaluating a brain tumor and planning therapy the neurosurgeon, however, has to classify the tumors according to certain biologic criteria.

Table 6. *"Clinical" Malignancy of Supratentorial Midline Tumors*

NEUROSURGICAL UNIVERSITY CLINIC VIENNA 1984 SUPRATENTORIAL MIDLINE TUMORS IN CHILDREN		
BENIGN	168	58 %
SEMIBENIGN	101	35 %
MALIGNANT	22	7 %
TOTAL	291	100 %

References

1. Brunner, C., cited in Rorschach, H., Zur Pathologie der Tumoren der Zirbeldrüse. Beitr. Klin. Chir. *83* (1913), 451.
2. Cairns, H., Mosberg, W. H., Jr., Colloid cyst of the third ventricle. Surg. Gynec. Obstet. *92* (1951), 545–570.
3. Camins, M. B., Schlesinger E. B., Treatment of tumours of the posterior part of the third ventricle and the pineal region: A long term follow-up. Acta Neurochir. (Wien) *40* (1978), 131–143.
4. Ciric, I., Zivin, I., Neuroepithelial (colloid) cysts of the septum pellucidum. J. Neurosurg. *43* (1975), 69–73.
5. Cummins, F. M., Taveras, J. N., Schlesinger E. B., Treatment of gliomas of the third ventricle and pinealomas. Neurology *10* (1960), 1031–1036.
6. Dandy, W. E., Benign Tumors in the Third Ventricle of the Brain. Diagnosis and Treatment, pp. 171. Springfield, Ill.: Ch. C Thomas. 1933.
7. Izquierdo, J. M., Rougerie, J., Lapras, C., Sanz, F., The so-called ectopic pinealomas—a cooperative study of 15 cases. Childs Brain *5* (1979), 505–512.
8. Jamieson, K. G., Excision of pineal tumors. J. Neurosurg. *35* (1971), 550–553.
9. Koos, W. T., Laubichler, W., Hirngeschwülste mit Beziehung zum Ventrikelsystem. Nervenarzt *35* (1964), 333–343.
10. Koos, W. T., Laubichler, W., Valencak, E., Les tumeurs du troisième ventricule chez l'enfant. Neuro-Chirurgie (Paris) *12* (1966), 645–652.
11. Koos, W. T., Geschwülste des Ventrikelsystems im Kindes- und Jugendalter. In: Pädiatrische Neurochirurgie (Kraus, H., Sunder-Plassmann, M., eds.), pp. 151–164. Wien: Wiener Med. Akademie. 1970.
12. Koos, W. T., Miller, M. H., Intracranial Tumors of Infants and Children. Stuttgart: Thieme. 1971.
13. Koos, W. T., Pendl, G., Zentrales und Peripheres Nervensystem. In: Krebsbehandlung als interdisziplinäre Aufgabe (Kärcher, K. H., ed.). Berlin-Heidelberg-New York: Springer. 1975.

14. Koos, W. T., Pendl, G., Die Tumoren des Zentralen Nerven-
systems. In: Chirurgische Onkologie (Denck, H., Karrer, K.,
eds.), pp. 563–582. Deerfield Beach, Fla.: Weinstein—Basel:
Edition Medizin. 1983.

15. Kraus, H., Koos, W. T., Hirntumoren im Kindes- und Jugendalter. Wiener Klin. Wschr. 79 (1967), 934–943.

16. Little, J. R., MacCarty, C. S., Colloid cysts of the third ventricle.
J. Neurosurg. 39 (1974), 230–235.

17. Rand, R. W., Lemmen, L. J., Tumors of the posterior portion of
the third ventricle. J. Neurosurg. 10 (1953), 1–18.

18. Rozario, R., Adelman, L., Prager, R. J., Stein, B. M.,
Meningiomas of the pineal region and third ventricle. Neurosurgery 5 (1979), 489–495.

19. Zülch, K. J., Biologie und Pathologie der Hirngeschwülste. In:
Handbuch der Neurochirurgie, Bd. 3 (Olivecrona, H., Tönnis,
W., eds.). Berlin-Göttingen-Heidelberg: Springer. 1956.

20. Zülch, K. J., Die Hirngeschwülste in biologischer und mor-
phologischer Darstellung, Third Edition. Leipzig: J. A. Barth.
1958.

21. Zülch, K. J., Die Pathologie und Biologie der Tumoren des
dritten Ventrikels. Acta Neurochir. (Wien) 9 (1961), 277–296.

22. Zülch, K. J., The present state of the classification of intracranial
tumors and its value for the neurosurgery. In: The Biology and
Treatment of Intracranial Tumors (Field and Sharkey, eds.), pp.
157–177. Springfield, Ill.: Ch. C Thomas. 1962.

23. Zülch, K. J., Die „Gradeinteilung" (Grading) der Malignität der
Hirngeschwülste. Acta Neurochir. (Wien) Suppl. 10 (1964), 639.

24. Zülch, K. J., Brain Tumors. Their Biology and Pathology, second
Edition. New York: Springer. 1965. Italian Edition: Padova:
Piccin Editors. 1974.

25. Zülch, K. J., Atlas of the Histology of Brain Tumors. Berlin-
Heidelberg-New York: Springer. 1971.

26. Zülch, K. J., Atlas of Gross Neurosurgical Pathology. Berlin-
Heidelberg-New York: Springer. 1975.

27. Zülch, K. J., Mennel, H. D., The biology of brain tumours.
Handbook of Clinical Neurology, Vol. 16. Amsterdam: North
Holland Publ. Comp. 1974.

Authors' address: Prof. Dr. W. T. Koos and Dr. A. Horaczek,
Department of Neurosurgery, University of Vienna Medical School,
Währinger Gürtel 18-20, A-1090 Wien, Austria.

Acta Neurochirurgica, Suppl. 35, 6–22 (1985)

B. Anatomy

Anatomy of the Midline

J. Lang

Institute of Anatomy, University of Würzburg, Federal Republic of Germany

Summary

Described are the anatomy and topography of the midline
structures particularly in relation to the surgical approaches.
Furthermore measurements of the third ventricle and the various
distances between surface areas of the brain and skull and different
landmarks of the cerebral midline are presented.

Keywords: Midline anatomy; sellar region; third ventricle; hypothalamus; pineal region; approaches.

Introduction

The midline structures of the brain lie in the central
part of the skull. Therefore all approaches to these
structures are relatively long. Various important brain
structures, nerves and vessels along these approaches
should be left undisturbed, if possible. In the following
pages these structures are described, as they are encountered along various routes.

Transnasal Approach to the Pituitary Region

In this approach the mucopereostium of the nasal
septum is displaced to reach the ostium of the sphenoid
sinus. Fig. 1 shows the dimensions of the nasal (piriform) aperture and its enlargement during postnasal
life. This bony structure is bordered superiorly by the
nasal bones and laterally and inferiorly by the maxilla,
including the premaxilla. The postnasal distance between the subspinous point and the aperture of the
sphenoid sinus is shown in Fig. 2, together with the
length of the anterior nasal spine (which may be
removed) and the distance between the subspinous
point and the nasal pores of the incisor canal (on both
sides of the nasal septum). Through this aperture the

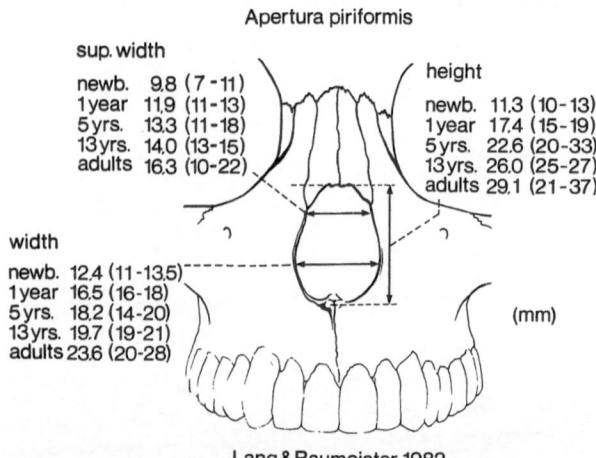

Fig. 1. Apertura piriformis, measurements of the superior width =
maximal distance of the lateral borders of the nasal bones, the
greatest width of the aperture and its height

medial branch of the greater palatine artery enters the
mucous membrane of the septum. This vessel forms a
plexus with the septal branches of the superior labial
artery (a twig of the facial artery), the anterior and
posterior ethmoidal arteries and the sphenopalatine
artery. The twigs of the latter have to be coagulated in
most cases along this approach (see Fig. 3). These
arteries reach the septum along the anteroinferior wall
of the sphenoid sinus.

The sinus is entered through its aperture, which is
located anterolaterally to the nasal septum and varies in
shape and size (see Lang 1983). The sinus appears in the
3rd to 4th months of fetal life. In one-year-old children
it has reached a length of about 7 mm and grows to
9 mm in the second and to 10 mm in the third year. By the

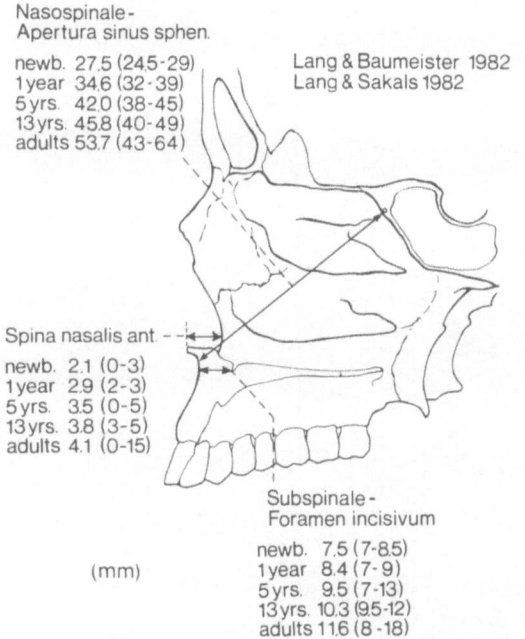

Nasospinale -
Apertura sinus sphen.

newb. 27.5 (24.5-29)
1 year 34.6 (32-39)
5 yrs. 42.0 (38-45)
13 yrs. 45.8 (40-49)
adults 53.7 (43-64)

Lang & Baumeister 1982
Lang & Sakals 1982

Spina nasalis ant.

newb. 2.1 (0-3)
1 year 2.9 (2-3)
5 yrs. 3.5 (0-5)
13 yrs. 3.8 (3-5)
adults 4.1 (0-15)

(mm)

Subspinale -
Foramen incisivum

newb. 7.5 (7-8.5)
1 year 8.4 (7-9)
5 yrs. 9.5 (7-13)
13 yrs. 10.3 (9.5-12)
adults 11.6 (8-18)

Fig. 2. Measurements of the nasospinal point (= paramedian point on the lowest border of the piriform aperture to the aperture of the sphenoidal sinus and the upper opening of the canalis incisivus

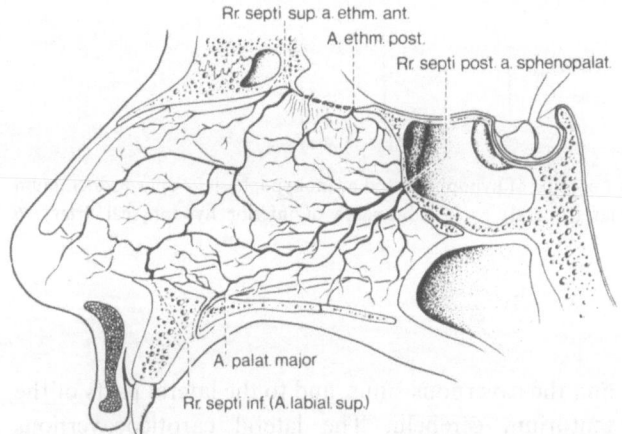

Rr. septi sup. a. ethm. ant.
A. ethm. post.
Rr. septi post. a. sphenopalat.
A. palat. major
Rr. septi inf. (A. labial. sup.)

Fig. 3. Main branches of the arteries of the septum nasi

fifth year it is 13 mm long and by the seventh it has attained a length of 20 mm. In adults we found the length of the sinus to measure 19.4 (6.5–32) mm in its superior part, 24.8 (9–36) mm in its central part and 18.5 (7–31) mm in its inferior part. Children have a relatively thick anterior-inferior bottom of the hypophyseal fossa, because pneumatization of the sphenoid bone occurs late.

According to Fujii *et al.* (1980) the average depth of the sphenoid sinus from the ostium to the nearest part

of the sella trucica is 17.1 (12.0–23.0) mm. This dimension is of surgical importance in the transnasal approach to the pituitary.

Location of the Pituitary in the Sella Turcica

During surgery the anterior lobe of the pituitary is yellowish and relatively firm, while the posterior lobe is gelatinous and gray. Hardy (1969) reported the anterior lobe to be surrounded by a potential cleft traversed by venous capillaries, which pass between the pituitary capsule and the periosteum of the sella turcica. The posterior lobe, by contrast, is usually firmly attached to the posterior wall of the pituitary fossa. We found much the same relationships in our material. Hardy (1969) saw numerous colloid follicles and venous capillaries within the intermediate lobe, which, for the purposes of surgical anatomy, mark the boundary between the anterior and posterior lobes. When the sphenoid sinus is of the sellar type, the dissector working from the sphenoid sinus outwards will find the periosteal layer of the dura to come into view after a thin layer of bone has been removed. The inferior intercavernous sinuses are incorporated in this periosteal layer. Next in line comes a potential cleft before the pituitary capsule is reached. Its inner surface is attached to the pituitary (Fig. 4).

Inferior Hypophyseal Artery and Capsular Artery

The inferior hypophyseal artery usually gives off small branches passing in the potential cleft between the pituitary capsule and the periosteal layer. Twigs of this vessel may reach the pituitary in a retrograde direction. Others pierce the floor of the sella turcica and contribute to the supply of the sphenoid bone and the mucoperiosteum of the sphenoid sinus.

Pituitary Adenomas and the "Empty Sella" (Fig. 5)

According to Domingue *et al.* (1978), pituitary adenomas sometimes occur in association with an "empty sella". The location of the hypophyseal cistern within the sella rarely gives any information on the site of a pituitary tumor. Domingue *et al.* (1978) state that the hypophyseal cistern was first described by Busch (1951) and later by Robertson (1967). Further studies of the "empty sella" and the hypophyseal cistern were made by Kaufman (1968) and Kaufman *et al.* (1972). Bergland *et al.* (1968) found a hypophyseal cistern in 20% of 225 autopsies. Domingue *et al.* (1978) found partially empty sellae in 17.3% of patients with amenorrhea and galactorrhea and in 10% of patients with acromegaly.

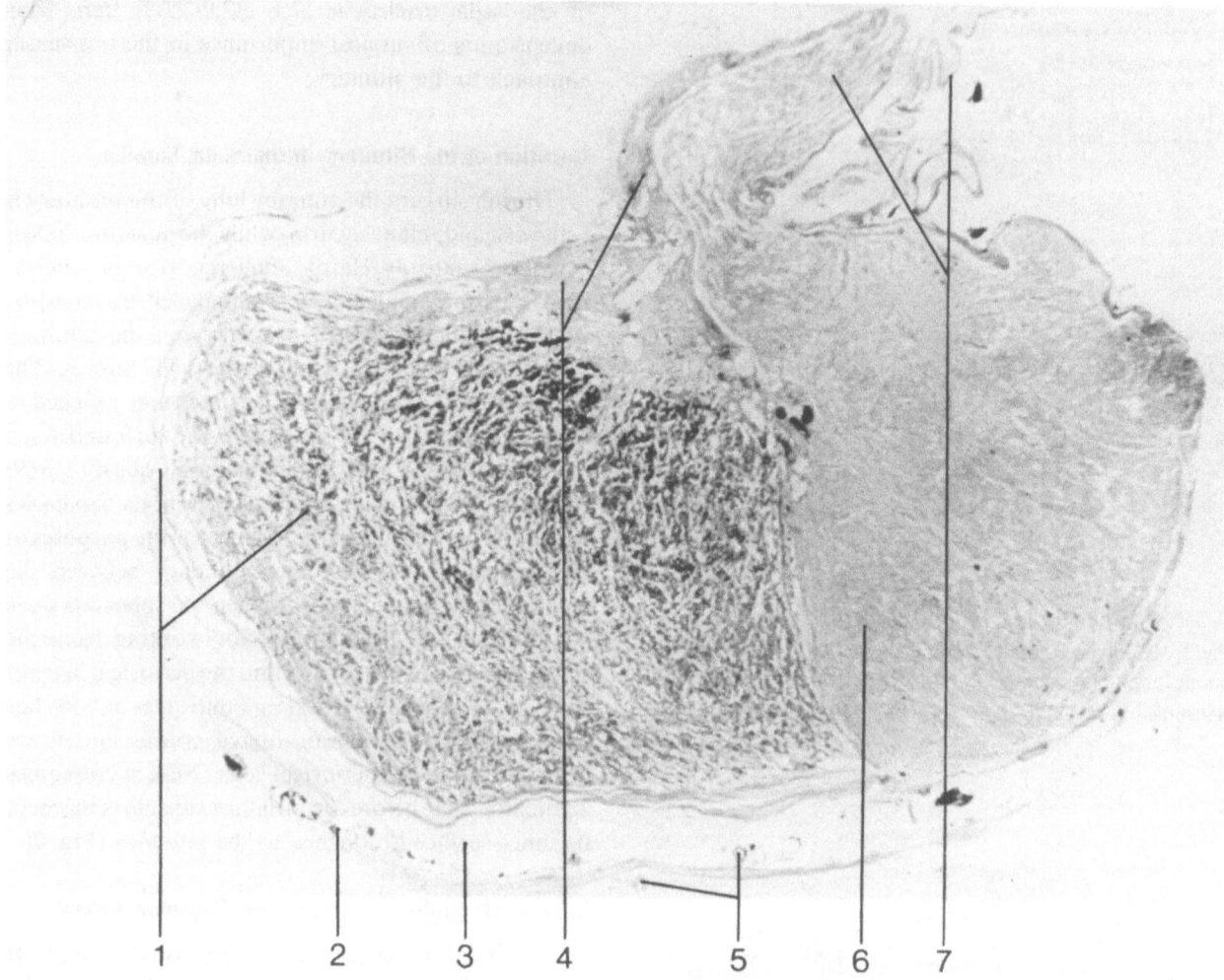

Fig. 4. Sagittal section of hypophysis surrounding connective tissue layers. *1* capsule of hypophysis and adenohypophysis; *2* dura-endocranium layer of pituitary fossa; *3* inferior intercavernous sinus; *4* infundibular (tuberal) part; *5* branches of inferior hypophyseal artery; *6* neurohypophysis; *7* infundibulum and arachnoïd membran

Caroticocavernous Trunks and Cavernous Sinus

In our material (Lang and Schäfer 1976) between 2 and 6 small arteries arose from the cavernous segment of the internal carotid artery. Most commonly there were two main trunks, which we termed the posterior and lateral caroticocavernous trunks. The posterior caroticocavernous trunk gives rise to the inferior hypophyseal artery to the pituitary fossa, and to twigs supplying the dura and bone of the dorsum sellae, the clivus, the perivascular tissue of the internal carotid artery and the carotid canal, the abducent nerve and the posterior surface of the temporal bone. There is also a superior caroticocavernous group which gives off fine branches to the anterior surface of the petrous part and the posterior surface, to the portal for the trigeminal nerve and the nerve itself, to the pars triangularis

and the cavernous sinus, and to the lateral parts of the tentorium cerebelli. The lateral caroticocavernous trunk may be between 1 and 4 mm long. It usually gives rise to the medial tentorial artery (marginal tentorial branch in the new nomenclature). This artery accompanies the trochlear nerve for some distance. It usually crosses the abducent nerve on the lateral side, but sometimes does so on the medial side, in which case it continues dorsally first into the transverse plate of the cavernous sinus and then below the trochlear nerve into the sagittal plate, fanning out and ramifying in the tentorium cerebelli, especially in the medial zones near the tentorial notch. Occasionally, this artery arises separtely from the sagittal segment of the internal carotid artery. In addition, this artery gives off small twigs to nerves III, IV and V, to the superior orbital

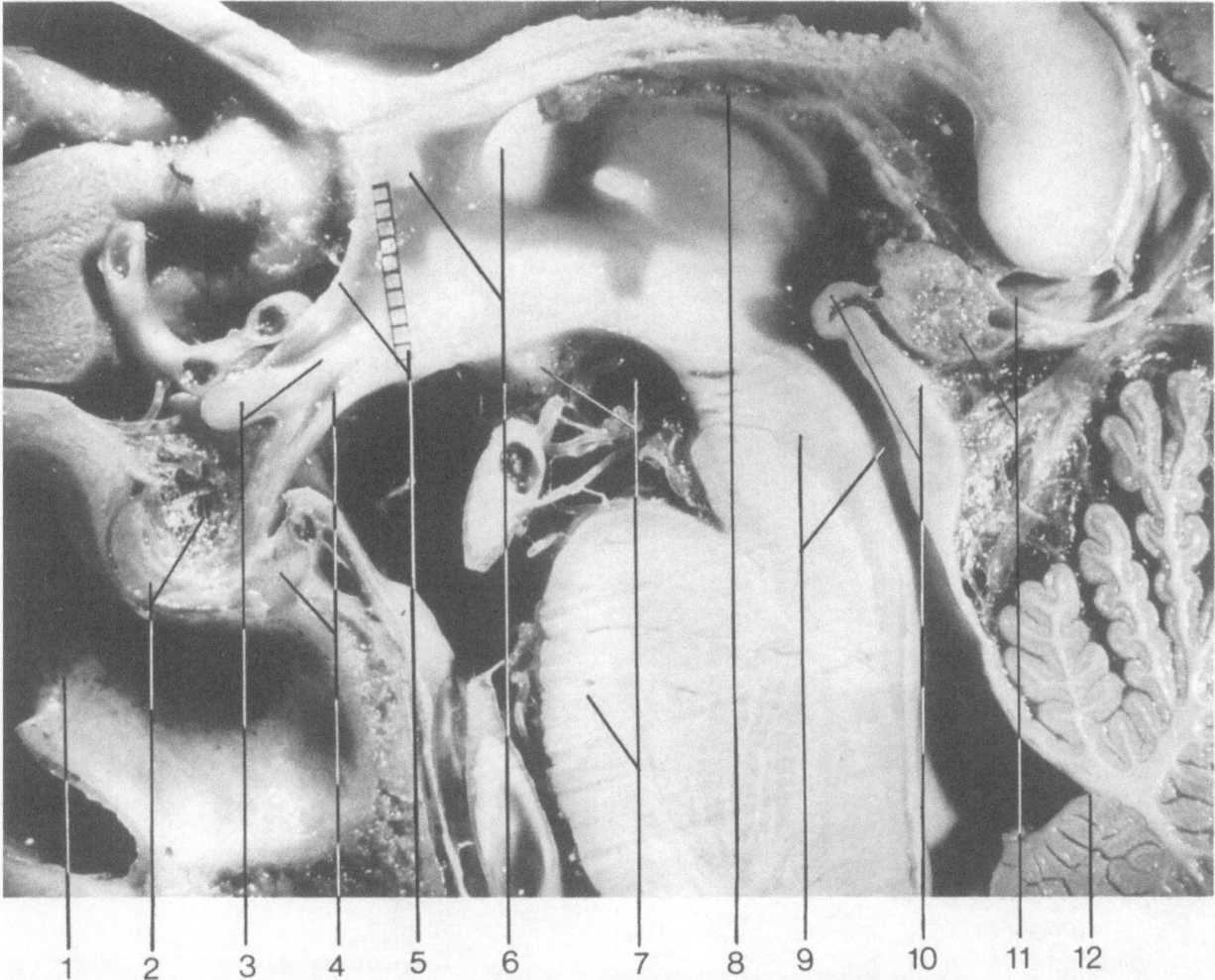

Fig. 5. "Empty sella", mediansagittal section, view from the left. *1* septum of sphenoidal sinus, oblique; *2* adenohypophysis, reduced and arachnoid tissue; *3* optic chiasm and chiasma point; *4* infundibular recess and neurohypophysis; *5* lamina terminalis, mm-paper; *6* rostral commissure and interventricular foramen; *7* mamillary body, interpeduncular fossa and pons; *8* choroid plexus of IIIrd ventricle; *9* tegmentum mesencephali and mesencephalic aqueduct; *10* epithalamic (posterior) commissure and lamina tecti; *11* pineal body and internal cerebral vein; *12* fastigium of IVth ventricle

fissure and to the bone and dura of the lesser wing of the sphenoid. Twigs for the abducent nerve, the anterior surface of the petrous bone and, occasionally, the middle and anterior-inferior hypophyseal arteries also arise from the lateral caroticocavernous trunk. These intracavernous branches of the internal carotid artery anastomose with one another and with twigs from the middle meningeal artery in the middle cranial fossa. They also anastomose with the meningeal branches of the vertebral artery, the ascending pharyngeal artery and other meningeal branches in the posterior cranial fossa.

Distance Between the Internal Carotid Arteries (Fig. 6)

Inside the cavernous sinus the two internal carotid arteries are separated by an average distance of 12 (4–18) mm between their medial walls. According to Renn and Rhoton jr. (1975) they may occasionally come as close as 4 mm.

The Pentagon

Hilal (1976) used the term pentagon to describe the median anterior basal cistern including the interpedun-

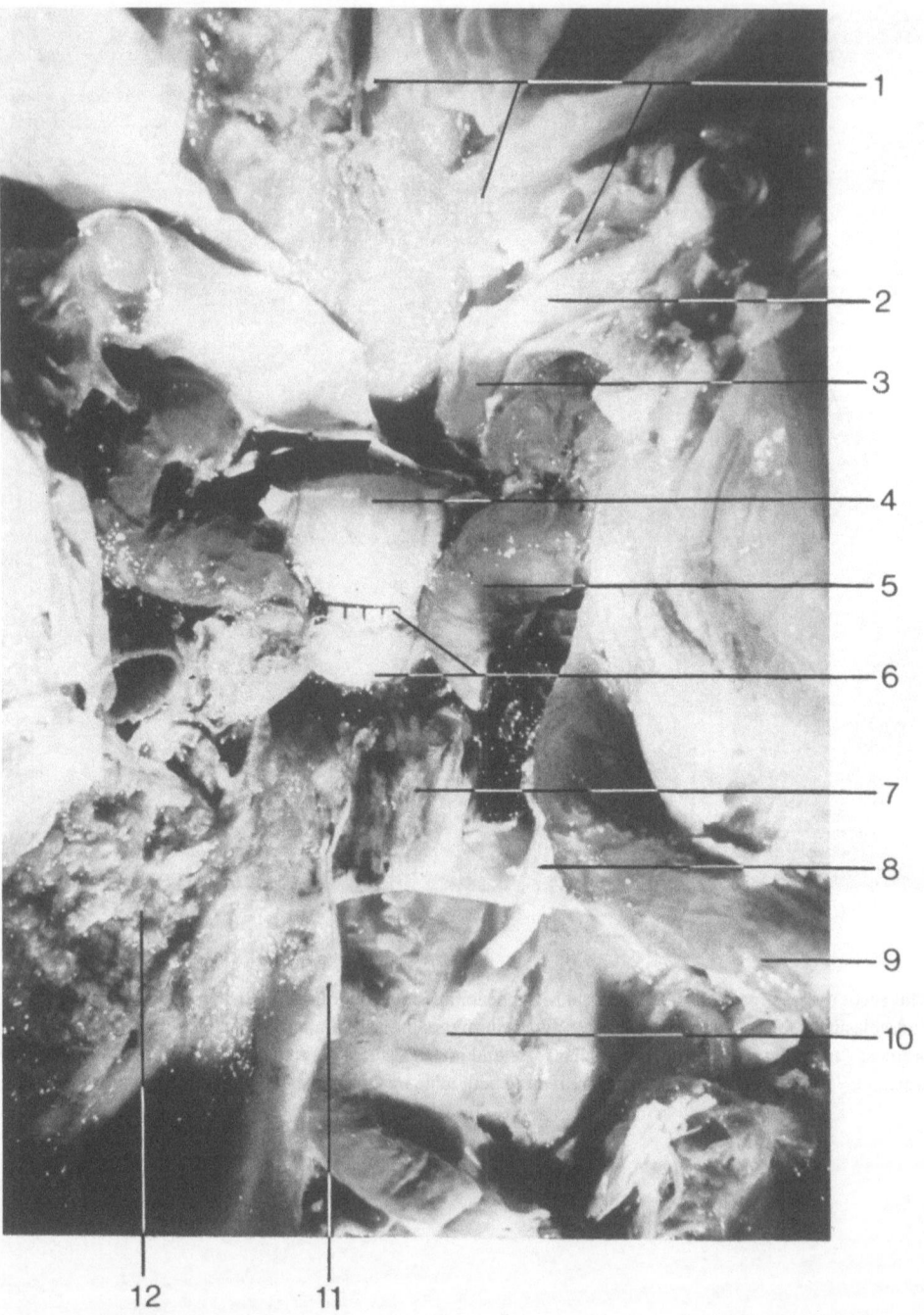

Fig. 6. Very short distance between both int. carotid arteries (viewed from caudally), spinal flood replaced by yellow gelatine. *1* dura mater, cut; *2* optic nerve, intracanalicular part; *3* intracranial part of optic nerve; *4* ant. lobe of hypophysis; *5* int. carotid artery; *6* mm-paper and posterior lobe of hypophysis; *7* dura mater of the clivus; *8* VIth nerve; *9* intracanalic. part of ICA; *10* subarachnoideal space of post. fossa; *11* dura mater of clivus; *12* petrous bone

cular cistern. This five-sided structure is usually demonstrable on the computer tomogram. It surrounds the pituitary stalk, the optic nerves and the optic chiasm and also includes the circle of Willis and the central branches of the latter. Its anterior boundary is formed by the posterior borders of the gyri recti, its lateral border by the uncus and parahippocampal gyrus, and its posterior border by the pons and the cerebral peduncles. Some arachnoid membranes divide the cistern in different compartments.

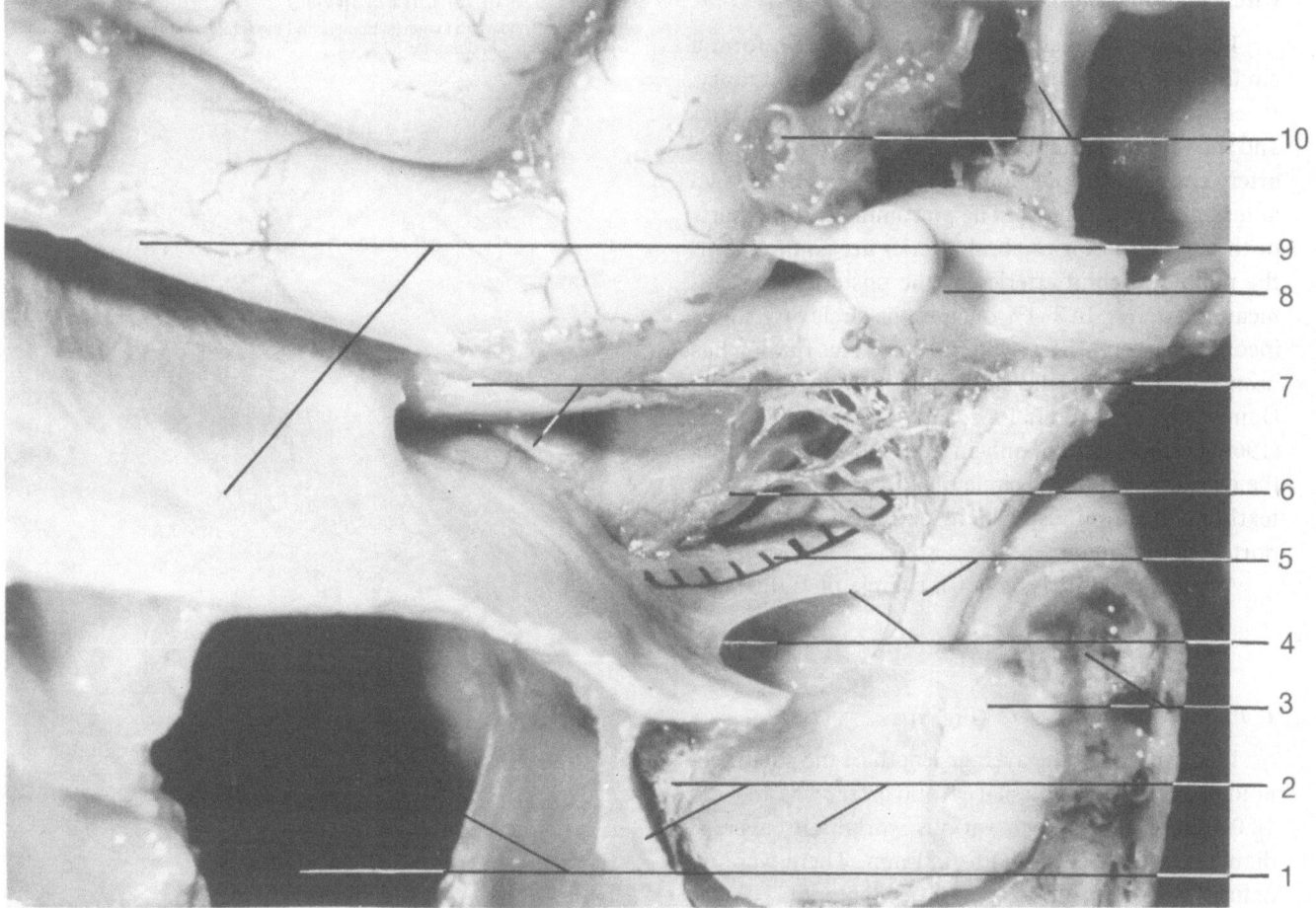

Fig. 7. Hypophyseal region, median sagittal section, viewed from the left. *1* sphenoidal sinus with oblique septum; *2* anterior intercavernous sinus and anterior wall of hypophyseal fossa and adenohypophysis; *3* neurohypophysis and dorsum selle; *4* diaphragmatic foramen, extremely large; *5* mm-paper and infundibulum; *6* superior hypophyseal artery with twigs to optic nerve and chiasma; *7* ophthalmic artery and optic nerve; *8* chiasma, displaced upwards with pin; *9* sphenoidal planum and gyrus rectus; *10* anterior communicating artery, cut, and lamina terminalis

Size of the Diaphragmatic Foramen (Fig. 7)

According to Bergland *et al.* (1968) the diaphragmatic foramen in old age has a diameter of 5 mm or more. Renn and Rhoton jr. (1975) found it to be round in 54% and transverse oval in 46%. With advancing age the infundibular orifice seems to enlarge. Besides the infundibulum, the superior hypophyseal arteries often pass through this foramen to reach the anterior lobe. Occasionally one of these arteries penetrates the diaphragm itself. Busch (1951), who examined no less than 788 pituitary regions and used the term operculum for the diaphragm, found it to be complete and to have a small opening for the pituitary stalk. The diaphragm is horizontal and consists of dense fibrous tissue. In 3.5% it has a funnel-shaped depression near the pituitary stalk.

Pituitary Cistern

The arachnoid invariably extends through the diaphragmatic foramen and spreads out onto the upper surface of the anterior lobe of the pituitary. In adults there is a fluid filled space within this arachnoid tissue, the pituitary cistern, which usually enlarges with advancing age. This cistern may extend anteriorly and laterally for a variable distance and may occasionally even overlap the posterior lobe. At the diaphragmatic foramen the arachnoid is always interwoven with the dura. This has prompted various workers to infer that the sellar diaphragm was composed of arachnoid (Shealey *et al.* 1968–in 65%). In the Würzburg material the pituitary cistern was clearly demonstrable in corrosion specimens. Bergland *et al.* (1968), using roentgenological methods, successfully demonstrated it inside the sella turcica in roughly 20% of cases.

Circle of Willis and Diencephalic Branches

The major arteries at the base of the brain form a circle within the pentagon, centered upon the pituitary. It receives blood from the two internal carotid arteries and the vertebral arteries. The anterior communicating artery connects the precommunicating parts of the two anterior cerebral arteries. The precommunicating parts of the two posterior cerebral arteries are connected to the middle cerebral arteries by the posterior communicating arteries. In 3–4% of cases the circle of Willis is incomplete (von Mitterwallner, 1955). This finding has been confirmed by the studies of later investigators (Jain 1964, Tseng and Li 1965, and others). McCormick (1969) pointed out that only in some 54% of cases does the development of the circle of Willis conform to the textbook descriptions. Alperg and Berry (1963) reported similar figures.

Affluents and divisions of the circle of Willis:

1. Internal Carotid Artery (Fig. 8)

In our material the average length of the subarachnoid segment of the internal carotid artery was 13.4 (8–18.0) mm. According to various workers its average diameter is 2.8–3.3 mm (1.6–3.8) mm. There were no definite right–left differences in our material.

2. Anterior Cerebral Artery

In our material the precommunicating part of the anterior cerebral artery averaged 13.5 (8–18.5) mm in length and 2.1 (0.75–3.75) mm in diameter. According to Wollschlaeger et al. (1967) hypoplastic arteries are present in approx. 8.6% (about 4% on the left and rather more than 3% bilaterally). These arteries have diameters of 1 mm or less. When the caliber of the anterior cerebral arteries is unusually narrow the main blood flow usually reaches the postcommunicating segment of the vessel via the anterior cerebral and anterior communicating arteries on the opposite side, both of which are correspondingly large. The precommunicating part of the artery is occasionally absent–in 1.1% (von Mitterwallner) or 0.7% (Krayenbühl and Yaşargil 1965).

3. Anterior Communicating Artery

In roughly 75% of cases the anterior communicating artery conforms to the textbook description (von

Cerebral arterial circle of Willis
Mean length and width in mm (extremes) and the fetal type of post.comm. art. More than 2mm in diameter 12%

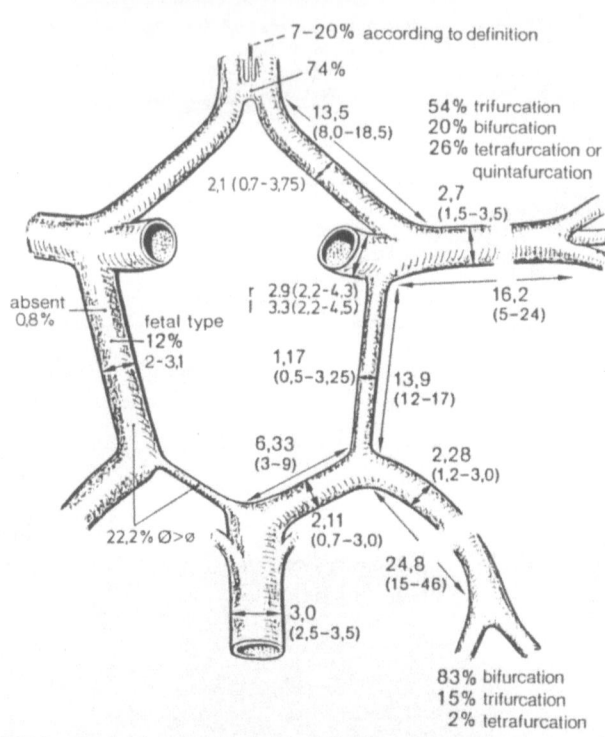

Fig. 8. Cerebral arterial circle of Willis with measurements of distances

Mitterwallner, 1955), but in approx. 9% it is reduplicated and V-shaped, Y-shaped or netlike in the remaining cases. RIGGS and RUPP (1963) found hypoplastic arteries in 9.3%. According to Perlmutter and Rhoton (1976) the average length of the anterior communicating artery is 2.6 (0.3–7.0) mm.

4. Middle Cerebral Artery

In our material the middle cerebral artery averaged 16.2 (5–24) mm in length and 2.7 (1.5–3.5) mm in diameter (Lang and Brunner 1978).

5. Posterior Communicating Artery

In our material the posterior communicating artery had an average length of 13.9 (12.0–17.0) mm and a diameter of 1.17 (0.5–3.25) mm. It is sometimes unusually large. If so it is regarded as being of the fetal type and provides the main inflow to the postcommunicating part of the posterior cerebral artery. In our material such fetal types made up 12%.

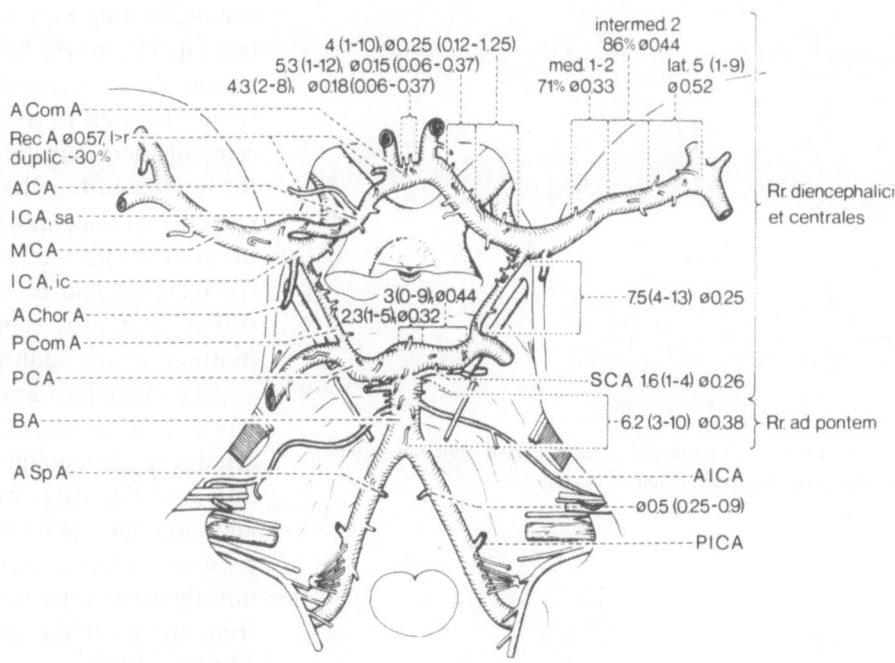

Fig. 9. Circulus arteriosus and its central rami, number and diameters

6. Precommunicating Part of the Posterior Cerebral Artery

In our material the precommunicating part of the posterior cerebral artery averaged 6.33 (3.0–9.0) mm in length and 2.11 (0.7–3.0) mm in diameter. When it is unusually narrow, the posterior communicating artery is usually of the fetal type.

Both the posterior communicating artery and the precommunicating part of the posterior cerebral artery may occasionally be absent.

7. Basilar Artery

The basilar artery supplies blood to the precommunicating parts of the posterior cerebral arteries. Its average diameter in our material was 3.0 (2.5–3.5) mm.

8. Central Branches of the Circle of Willis (Fig. 9)

The central branches of the circle of Willis are of clinical importance not only because of the territories they supply, but also because of the occurence of basal aneurysms at their origins. Among the structures supplied by these branches, the most important is the diencephalon.

Anterior Choroidal Artery

In our material the anterior choroidal artery arose from the internal carotid artery in 96%; in 2% it was a branch of the posterior communicating artery and in another 2% it had a double origin from both of these vessels. Its point of origin is 2.9 (0.5–5) mm proximal to the division of the internal carotid artery (Brunner 1978). The vessel has an average diameter of 0.77 (0.4–1.25) mm. It courses posteriorly along the lower and lateral surface of the optic tract and passes into the temporal horn of the lateral ventricle through the choroid fissure. Along the course it gives off numerous twigs to the diencephalon.

Inferior Diencephalic Branches (Fig. 10)

Even in the latest Nomina Anatomica (1977) the subclassification of the branches of the circle of Willis at the base of the brain is extremely inconsistent. Vessels arising from the anterior cerebral and anterior communicating arteries and entering the diencephalon are designated as anteromedial central arteries and branches; to those are added the anterolateral central arteries from the middle cerebral artery and the posteromedial central arteries and thalamic branches from the posterior cerebral artery.

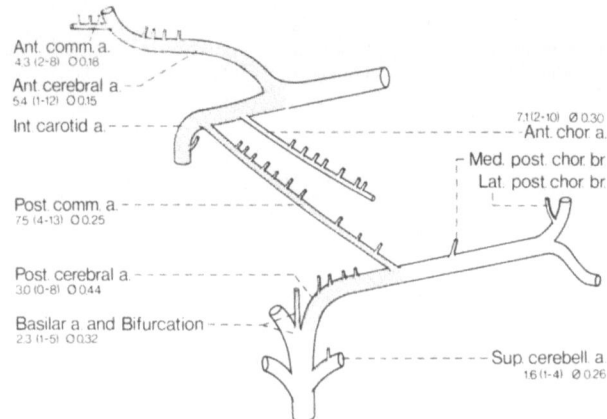

Fig. 10. Inferior diencephalic branches from different arteries, number (extremals) and diameter (mean)

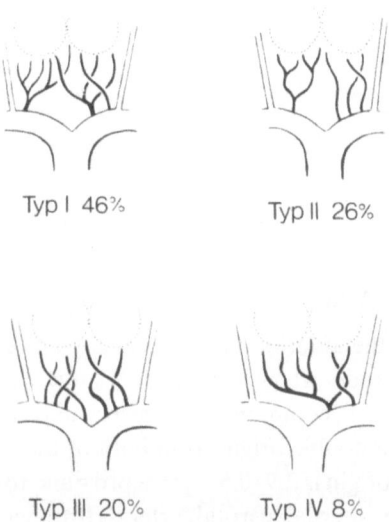

Typ I 46%   Typ II 26%

Typ III 20%   Typ IV 8%

Rami diencephalici inferiores posteriores

Fig. 11. Different origin and course of the rami diencephalici inferiores posteriores with origin of the p_1 segment (Brunner 1978)

In Nomina Anatomica a further subdivision is made for the twigs of the anterior choroidal artery (rami to optic tract, lateral geniculate body, internal capsule, globus pallidus, tuber cinereum, hypothalamic nuclei, etc.). Before the publication of these Nomina we suggested that the diencephalic vessels, which arise from the anterior cerebral and anterior communicating arteries, should be named anterior inferior diencephalic branches, and proposed the terms inferior diencephalic branches for the vessels arising from the posterior communicating artery, and posterior inferior diencephalic branches for those arising from the pre-

communicating part of the posterior cerebral artery (see Fig. 11), for the basilar and the superior cerebellar arteries the term lateral inferior diencephalic branches should be used to denote the twigs from the middle cerebral artery, which contribute to the blood supply of the anterior parts of the diencephalon, and those arising from the anterior choroidal artery and perfuse mainly the posterior parts of the diencephalon. The latter enter the diencephalon at various points along its lower surface and also supply other parts of the brain (portions of the midbrain and telencephalon).

The mamillary arteries are not listed in the new Nomina anatomica. On an average there are three arteries to the mamillary body, each of which divides into 3–12 fine twigs with diameters of 0.05–0.15 mm and forms an arterial rate. The affluents arise from the posterior inferior diencephalic branches (in 47%), directly from the posterior cerebral artery (in 29%) and from the posterior communicating artery (in 24%) (Brunner 1978).

Frontal and Frontolateral Approach to the Pituitary Region

The length, course, width and central branches of the *anterior cerebral artery* are of clinical importance in the surgical approach to the pituitary region from the frontal or the anterolateral aspects. In our material the length of the subarachnoid segment of the internal carotid artery was 13.65 (10–18) mm on the right and 13.14 (8–18) mm on the left. The artery courses posteriorly and then dorsolaterally, giving off the anterior cerebral artery from its anterior circumference in 61.8% and from its superior circumference in 38.2% of cases (Firbas and Sinzinger 1972). The precommunicating part of the anterior cerebral artery has an average length of 13.5 mm and an average width of 2.1 mm and runs medially and forward above the optic nerve or chiasm. It then gives off the anteromedial central arteries (anteromedial thalamostriate arteries), which continue backward and laterally to the anterior perforated substance. Arising further distally, close to the anterior communicating artery, there are smaller twigs to the inferior anterior regions of the midbrain. We have termed these the anterior inferior diencephalic rami (Lang and Brunner 1978). Together with direct branches from the internal carotid artery, they supply the optic nerve, optic chiasm, lamina terminalis, optic tract, and the anterior inferior parts of the diencephalon. Separate twigs course upward to the small anterior segment of the caudate nucleus. The paraventricular, dorsomedial, preoptic, supraoptic and tuberal nuclei are supplied by these twigs, as are the anterior portion of the infundibulum and the lateral wall of the third ventricle as far as the interventricular foramen and the anterior commissure. There are also inferior and anterior diencephalic branches, averaging 4.26 in number, which arise from the anterior communicating artery and supply these regions (Fig. 22).

Long central artery (anterior recurrent artery, Heubner's artery): The origin of the long central artery, which likewise courses to the anterior perforated substance, lies from 8 mm proximal to 3 mm distal to the origin of the anterior communicating artery from the anterior cerebral artery. On an average, it is 0.4 mm distal to the anterior communicating artery; this is its site of origin in approximately 60% of cases. In approx. 30% the artery arises at the level of the anterior communicating artery; an origin proximal to it was only seen in 11.3% (Lang and Brunner 1978). In our material the long recurrent artery was duplicated in about 30% of cases, a triple artery was present in about 1%.

The average diameter of the long central artery is 0.57 (0.31–0.87) mm. On the left side the vessel is somewhat wider (0.60 mm) than on the right (0.54 mm), this difference being statistically significant. In roughly twothirds of cases the artery has branches which contribute to the supply of the olfactory bulb, olfactory tract and the orbital part of the frontal lobe. The artery runs backward and laterally in close proximity to the anterior cerebral artery, crosses the latter approximately 15 mm distal to its origin and usually penetrates the anteromedial region of the anterior perforated substance (Kollmannsberger 1961).

Anterior communicating artery: As a rule, the two anterior cerebral arteries are connected by a short trunk (anterior communicating artery) situated above the optic chiasm in 70% according to Perlmutter and Rhoton jr. 1976. In 30% of cases the anterior communicating artery lies at the level of the optic nerves and 5–30 mm above the sphenoid plane (angiographic studies by Krayenbühl and Yaşargil 1965). There are numerous morphological variants.

The medial frontobasal branch (medial frontobasal artery) (Fig. 13) of the anterior cerebral artery runs forward and basally along the medial surface of the hemisphere towards the frontal pole. Several twigs of this artery curve round the medial inferior edge of the hemisphere and supply the orbital part of the frontal

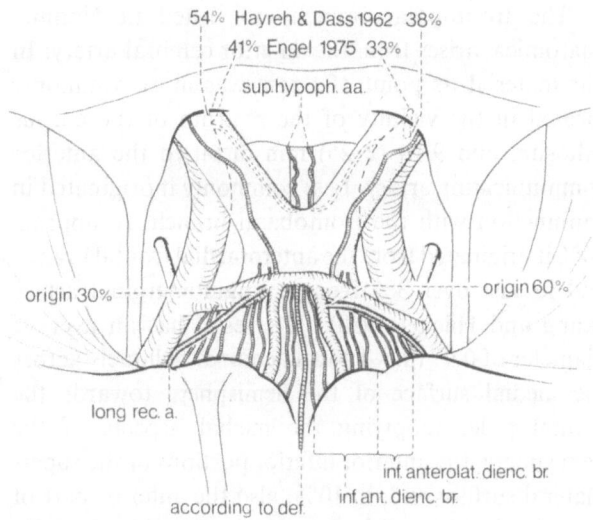

Fig. 12. Arteries of the hypophyseal region by frontal or frontolateral approaches (the most common course of the ophthalmic artery and its origin, vessels to the upper surface of the optic nerve and chiasm, Heubner's artery, different origins, inferior diencephalic branches and anterior median cerebral artery)

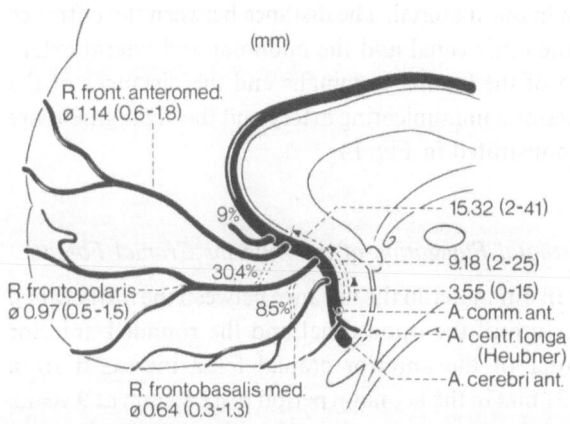

Fig. 13. Branches of the anterior cerebral artery to the medial lower surface of the forebrain, diameter (extremals), origin zones measured to the anterior communicating artery in mm (extremals)

lobe from its medial side. In our material (100 hemispheres) the artery usually arose from the anterior cerebral artery at a point roughly 3.55 (0–15) mm distal to the anterior communicating artery; in approx. 8.5% it originated from the frontopolar branch, in 8.5% from the anteromedial frontal branch and in 1% from the long central artery. Reduplication of the medial frontobasal branch is not uncommon, and sometimes it courses on the orbital surface of the frontal lobe (Lang and Häckel 1980).

The frontopolar branch, not listed in Nomina anatomica, arises from the anterior cerebral artery: In our material its point of origin was most commonly located in the vicinity of the rostrum of the corpus callosum and 9.18 (2–25) mm distal to the anterior communicating artery. Less commonly it originated in conjunction with the frontobasal branch. In approx. 30% it originated from the anteromedial frontal branch and in just over 3% from a cingulomarginal artery (Lang and Häckel 1980). The vessel has an average diameter of 0.97 (0.5–1.5) and courses obliquely across the medial surface of the hemisphere towards the frontal pole, supplying the medial aspects of the hemisphere, the anterior inferior portions of the superolateral surface and, in 10%, also the anterior part of the orbital surface of the frontal lobe. Combined supply of this area from the contralateral artery has been observed.

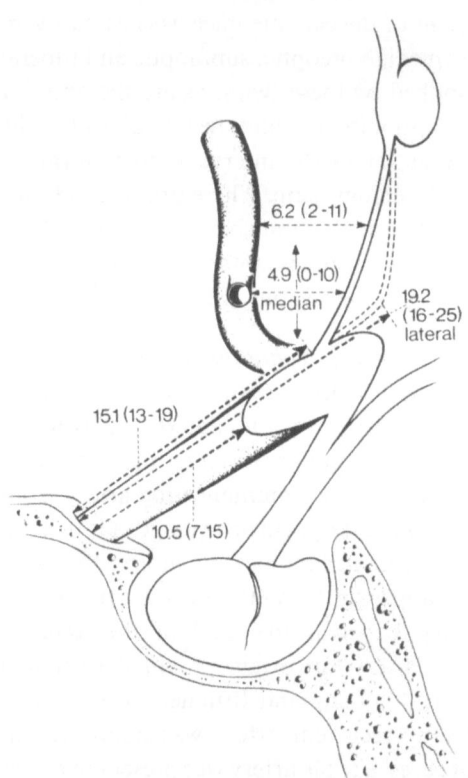

Fig. 14. Measurements between the intracranial (dural) opening of the optic canal to the chiasm, median lower part of lamina terminalis, lateral part of lamina terminalis and distances between the anterior communicating artery and lamina terminalis and the A_2 segment and lamina terminalis

Distance from the Optic Canal

The medial length of the optic nerve was 10.5 (7–15) mm in our material. The distance between the entrance in the optic canal and the midpoint and lateral extension of the lamina terminalis and the distances of the anterior communicating artery and the A2 segment are demonstrated in Fig. 14.

Postnatal Elongation of the Anterior Cranial Fossa

In our material the distance between the intracranial aperture of the optic canal and the rounded anterior border of the anterior cranial fossa increased from 29.31 mm in the neonatal period to 42.83 mm at 9 years. In adults the average distance is about 45 (36–54) mm (Fig. 15).

On the basis of X-ray studies Stramrud (1959) reported an uncorrected distance (0–5.6%) between the inner table of the frontal bone and the midpoint of the hypophyseal fossa of 53.2 mm in 3-year-old children. At 6 years this distance was 56.9 mm and in adults it had reached 57.3 mm (mean values).

Postnatal Changes of Cribiform Plate

Up to 9 years of age the cribiform plate grows in length; thereafter that part of it which is visible from above shortens again to approximately the same size as in the newborn. This is due to the fact that the sphenoid plane overgrows the posterior part of the ethmoid bone

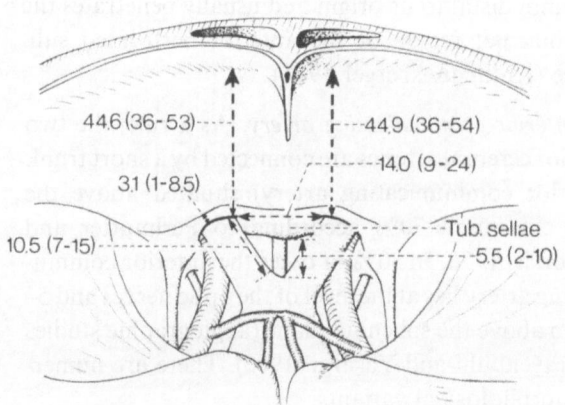

Fig. 15. Distances of different structures of the hypophyseal region: from the inner surface of the lowest part of the squama frontalis to the dural opening of the optic canal, length of the dural covering of the optic canal (shown on the left), distance between the medial borders of the optic nerve, medial length of the optic nerve and distance between tuberculum sellae and chiasm. Measurements in mm (extremals)

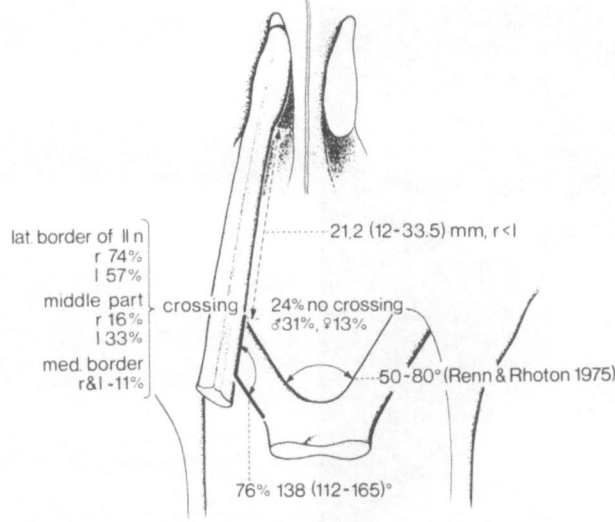

Fig. 16. Length of the olfactory tract between olfactory bulb and crossing zone with optic nerve. No crossing occurs on our material in 24%. Given is also the angle between the two optic nerves according to Renn and Rhoton (1975)

from behind, the part chiefly involved being its anteriorly projecting middle portion, which is also known as the ethmoidal spine of the sphenoid bone (Schmidt 1975). Until adulthood the width of the cribiform plate decreases by 1.6 mm in its anterior segments, while the posterior segments become slightly (by 0.5 mm) wider. Schmidt (1975) believed the narrowing of the anterior segments to be due to thickening of the crista galli and probably also to the increased pneumatization of the ethmoid air cells.

Formation of the Olfactory Fossa

According to Schmidt (1975) the average vertical distance between the medial endofrontal fovea and the cribiform plate is approximately 5 mm during perinatal life and decreases somewhat up to age 9 years, but has increased again by approximately 6 mm by the time adulthood is reached.

Distance Between the Prechiasmal Groove and Tuberculum Sellae

In adults the anterior border of the prechiasmal groove is marked by a transverse ridge which extends between the two intracranial apertures of the optic canals and is also visible on the dura. In our material the average distance between this dural fold and the tuberculum sellae was 6.8 (3.3–10.3) mm (Lang and Haas 1979).

The length of the anterior border of the prechiasmal groove (jugum sphenoidale and the posterior border of the cribiform plate) increases in length from 7.5 mm in newborns to 10.42 mm in 9-year-old children to 14.19 mm by adults (mean values). The area is in my view the mean growth center of the anterior fossa bottom region.

Fig. 16 shows the angle between the olfactory tract and the optic nerve.

Pterional Approach

The pterion is the sutural zone between the frontal bone, the greater wing of the sphenoid, the parietal

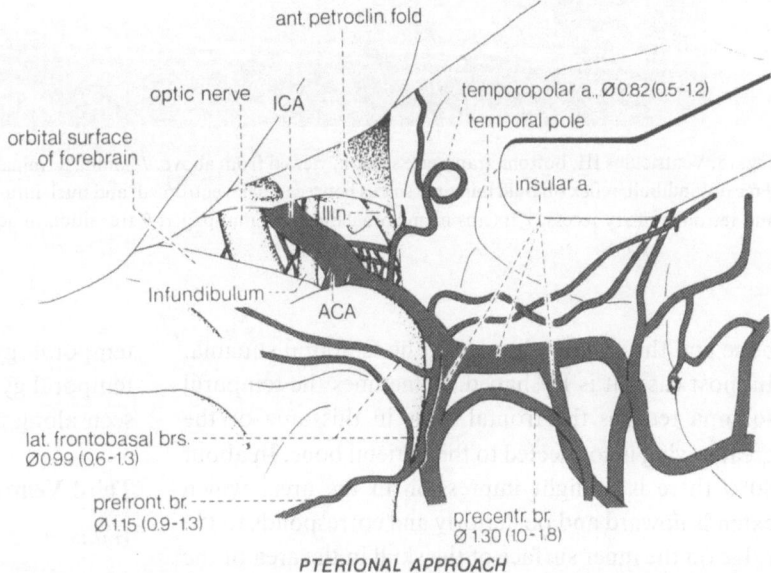

Fig. 17. Vessels and nerves which are seen by pterional approach to the hypophyseal region, some measurements of different branches of the middle cerebral artery are given, in mm (extremals)

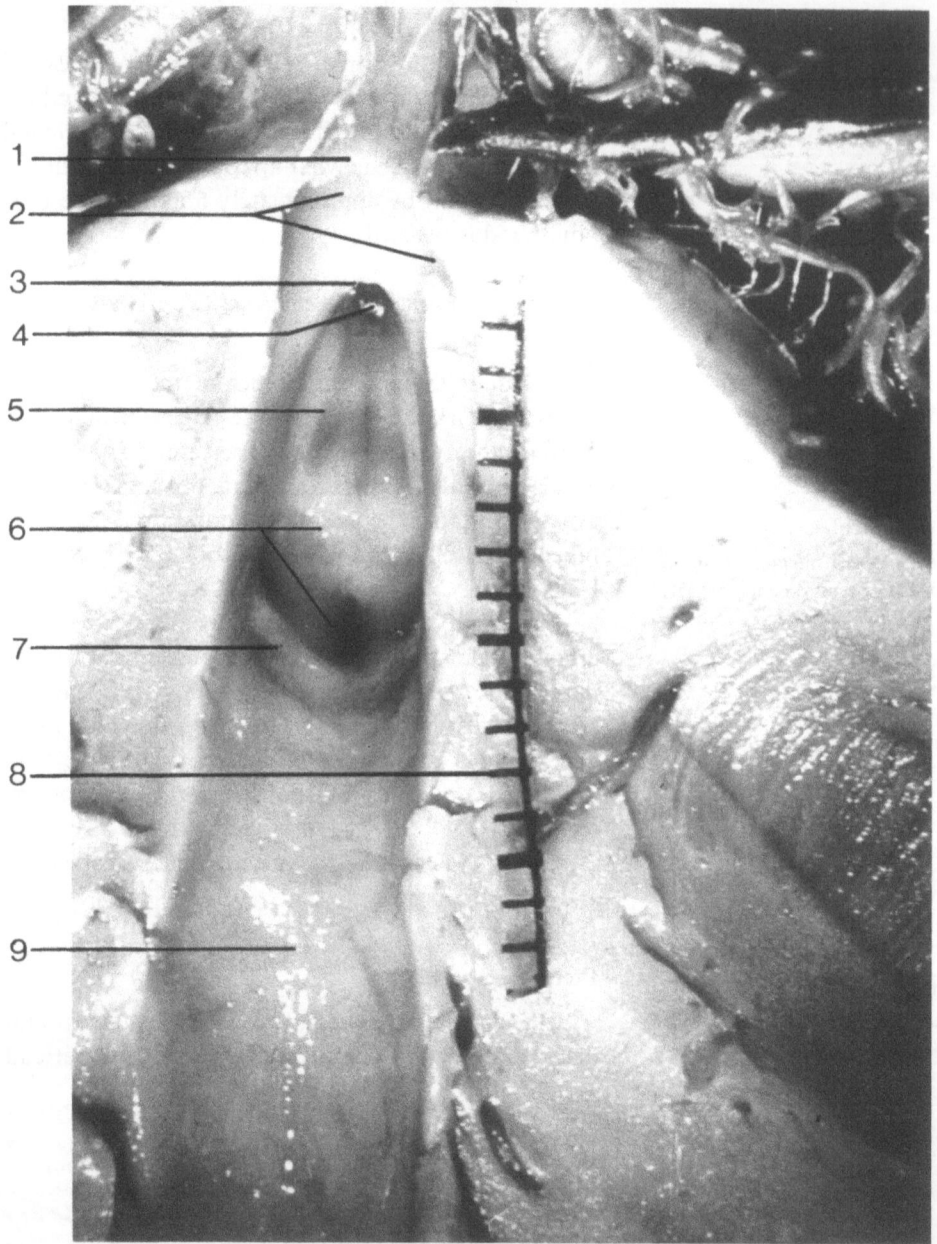

Fig. 18. Ventriculus III, bottom, transverse section, viewed from above. *1* lamina terminalis; *2* rec. opticus, anterior and lateral parts; *3* chiasm; *4* rec. infundibuli, reflex on fluid mirror; *5* sulcus between nucl. ventromed. and nucl. infundibularis (arcuatus); *6* corpus mamillare, prominence and retromamillary recess; *7* tractus mamillothalamicus; *8* mm-paper; *9* transition in aqueductus mesencephali

bone and the anterior border of the temporal squama. In most cases it is H-shaped. Sometimes the temporal squama reaches the frontal bone in this area or the greater wing is connected to the parietal bone. In about 80% there is a slight impression in the area, which extends upward and posteriorly and corresponds to the ridge on the inner surface of the skull in the area of the lateral cerebral sulcus. Below this impression a protuberance is often felt. It corresponds to the superior temporal gyrus, more often to one of the middle temporal gyruses below it. In Fig. 17 the main arteries seen along the pterional approach are shown.

Third Ventricle

Walls

The anterior wall of the third ventricle is formed in its upper part by the anterior commissure. Proceeding

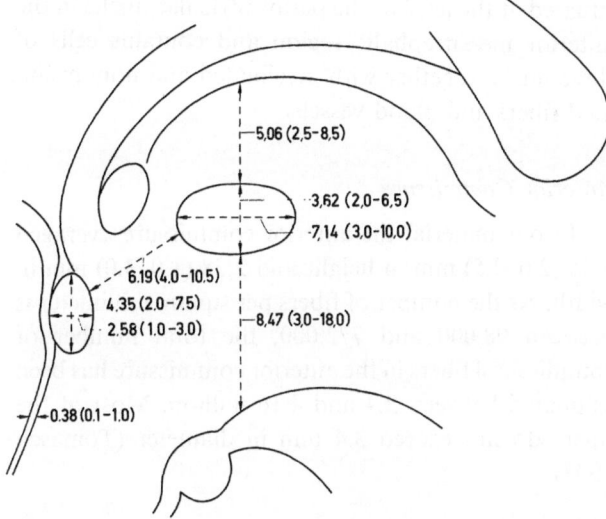

Fig. 19. Measurements of the rostral commissure, the interthalamic adhesion and the lamina terminalis and distances between the structures and roof and bottom of the IIIrd ventricle, in mm (extremals)

forward and downward, we next come to the thin lamina terminalis, which also forms the anterior wall of the optic recess. Immediately behind it the optic chiasm rises from below into the third ventricle for a variable distance and forms the posterior wall of the optic recess. Dorsal to the transverse spur of the chiasmal region the cavity of the third ventricle descends as the infundibulum into the pituitary stalk. From the posterior wall of the latter the floor ascends backward and upward over the mamillary bodies to the interpeduncular perforated substance and the aqueduct of the midbrain. The epithalamic (posterior) commissure is situated above the entry to the aqueduct. Between the habenulae is the pineal recess and above the pineal body is the suprapineal recess. The roof of the third ventricle is lined by ependyma which is covered by, and adherent to, a layer of pia mater, named the tela choroidea of the third ventricle. The tela extends forward as far as the posterior border of the interventricular foramen. The folds and villi of the choroid plexus of the third ventricle project from it even in fetal life. For further details see Lanz/Wachsmuth, Praktische Anatomie, Vol. 1, 1 A. The bottom of the third ventricle is shown in Fig. 18.

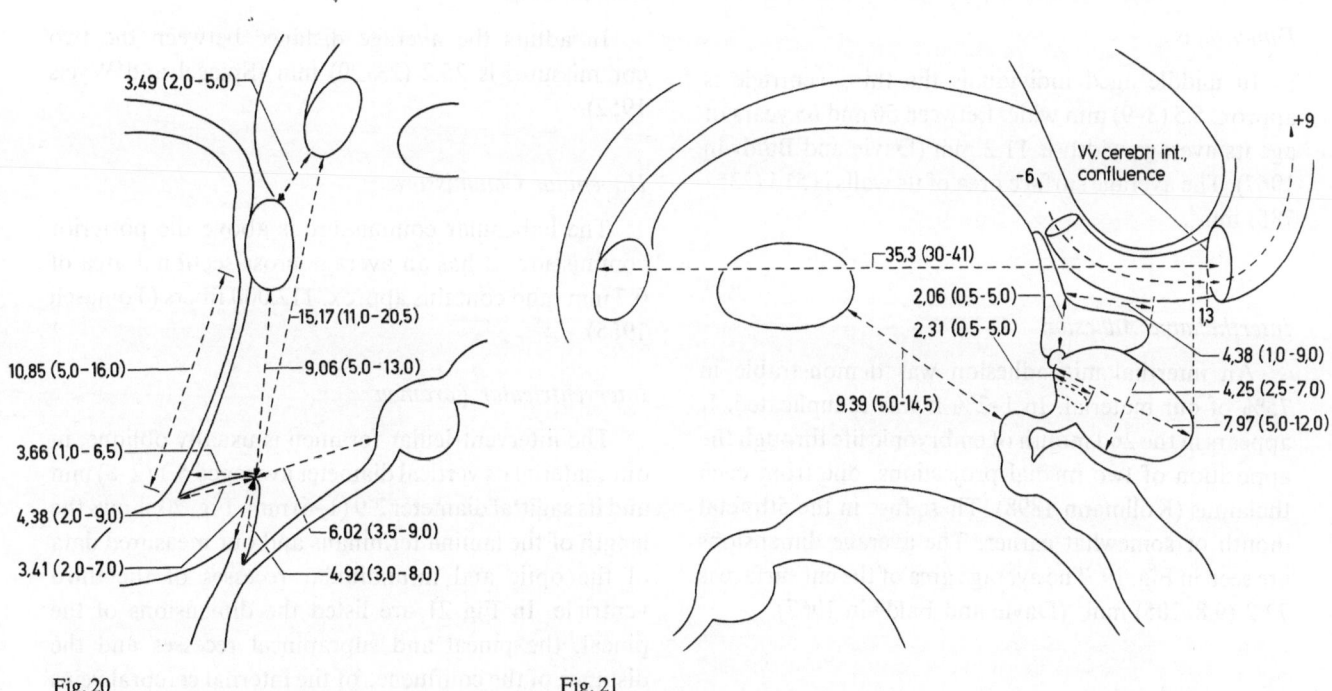

Fig. 20   Fig. 21

Fig. 20. Distances of structures of the anterior part of the IIIrd ventricle, between the rostral commissure and foramen interventriculare, length of the lamina terminalis, distances from the lower border of the rostral commissure and the foramen interventriculare to the chiasm point and entrance and depth of the optic and infundibular recesses, in mm (extremals)

Fig. 21. Measurements of the posterior part of the IIIrd ventricle and neighboring structures (confluence) of internal cerebral veins to anterior border of foramen interventriculare, length and height of the suprapineal and pineal recesses, height and length of the pineal body and distance between the interthalamic adhesion and epithalamic (posterior) commissure, in mm (extremals)

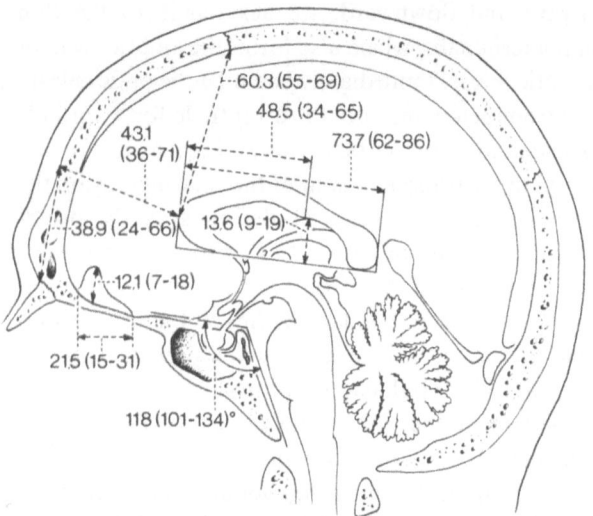

Fig. 22. Measurements for different aproaches to the IIIrd ventricle. Given are the height of the crista galli and its length, the shortest distance between the genu corporis callosi and the outer surface of the skull and the height above the nasion, distance between the bregma and the genu of corpus callosi, length of the corpus callosum and the zone of attachement of the fornix to corpus callosum and its height above the basal line of corpus callosum. Shown is also the angle between the planum sphenoidale and the clivus in adults. All measurements in mm (extremals and degrees)

Dimensions

In middle aged individuals the third ventricle is approx. 5.5 (3–9) mm wide. Between 56 and 65 years of age its average width is 11.2 mm (Davie and Baldwin 1967). The average surface area of its walls is 515 (235–785) mm².

Interthalamic Adhesion

An interthalamic adhesion was demonstrable in 75% of our material. In 1–2% it was reduplicated. It appears in the 2nd month of embryonic life through the apposition of two medial projections, one from each thalamus (Kollmann 1898). These fuse in the 5th fetal month or somewhat earlier. The average dimensions are seen in Fig. 19. The average area of the cut surface is 72.2 (9.8–205) mm² (Davie and Baldwin 1967).

Third Ventricle and Surrounding Structures

Supraoptic Commissure

Van der Rahe (1937) found a supraoptic commissure (of Ganser) to be present in 2.15% in front of the interthalamic adhesion and often below it as well. It is

situated at the level of the paraventricular nuclei in the anterior mesencephalic region and contains cells of these nuclei together with myelinated and nonmyelinated fibers and blood vessels.

Anterior Commissure

In our material the anterior commissure averaged 4.35 (2.0–7.5) mm in height and 2.58 (1.0–3.0) mm in width. As the number of fibers per square millimeter is between 98,000 and 772,000, the total number of commissural fibers in the anterior commissure has been estimated between 2.4 and 4.16 million. Most of the fibers do not exceed 3.4 mm in diameter (Tomasch 1957).

Epithalamic (Posterior) Commissure

The posterior commissure has an average cut surface area of 3.58 mm² and contains between 497,000 and one million fibers. According to Spiegel and Wycis (1952) its average distance from the center of the interthalamic adhesion is 14.8 (13.5–16.0) mm.

Distance Between the Anterior and Posterior Commissures

In adults the average distance between the two commissures is 25.2 (23–29) mm (Spiegel and Wycis 1952).

Habenular Commissure

The habenular commissure is above the posterior commissure. It has an average cross-sectional area of 0.7 mm² and contains approx. 112,000 fibers (Tomasch 1965).

Interventricular Foramen

The interventricular foramen is usually oblique; in our material its vertical diameter averaged 5.1 (2–8) mm and its sagittal diameter 2.9 (1–6) mm. Fig. 20 shows the length of the lamina terminalis and our measured data of the optic and infundibular recesses of the third ventricle. In Fig. 21 are listed the dimensions of the pineal, the pineal and suprapineal recesses and the distance of the confluence of the internal cerebral veins and the anterior border of the foramen of Monro. Figs. 22 and 23 show our measured distances (on median and paramedian sagittal sections) of different points of the corpus callosum from the outer and inner surfaces of the skull. Also shown are length in supra- and infratentorial approaches to the pineal region.

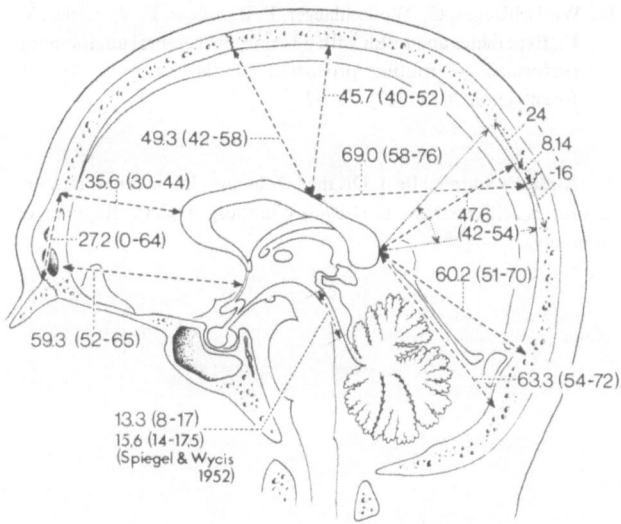

Fig. 23. Measurements betweeen the inner surface of the skull to lamina terminalis, genu corporis callosi, truncus corporis callosi and the shortest distance between the splenium and the lambda (situated in the mean 8.14 mm anterior to lambda) and distances between the splenium corporis callosi above and below of the tentorium cerebelli 1 cm paramedian. Included are measurements of Spiegel and Wycis (1952) for the length of the aqueduct, our measurements [13.3. (8-17) mm] belong to the lamina tecti. All measurements in mm (extremals)

References

1. Alpers, B. J., Berry, R. G., Circle of Willis in cerebral vascular disorders. Arch. Neurol. *8* (1963), 398–402.
2. Bergland, R., Ray, B., Torack, R., Anatomical variations in the pituitary gland and adjacent structures in 225 human autopsy cases. J. Neurosurg. *28* (1968), 93–99.
3. Brunner, F. K., Über die Arterien des Hirnstammes, Vorkommen, Zahl, Durchmesser und Variationen. Med. Diss. (Würzburg) (1978).
4. Busch, W., Die Morphologie der Sella turcica und ihre Beziehung zur Hypophyse. Virchows Archiv für pathologische Anatomie und Physiologie und für klinische Medizin *320* (1951), 437–458.
5. Davie, J. C., Baldwin, M., Radiographic anatomical study of the massa intermedia. J. Neurosurg. *26* (1967), 483–487.
6. Domingue, J. N., Wing, S. D., Wilson, C. B., Coexisting pituitary adenomas and partially empty sellas. J. Neurosurg. *48* (1978), 23–28.
7. Firbas, W., Sinzinger, H., Über den Anfangsteil der Arteria cerebri anterior. Acta Anat. *83* (1972), 81–86.
8. Fujii, K., Lenkey, C., Rhoton, A. L., Microsurgical anatomy of the choroidal arteries. Fourth ventricle and cerebellopontine angles. J. Neurosurg. *52* (1980), 504–524.
9. Hardy, J., Transphenoidal microsurgery of the normal and pathological pituitary. Clin. Neurosurg. *16* (1969), 185–217.
10. Hilal, S. K., CT in evaluation of orbital disease. Int. Symposium: Computed Cranial Tomography. Hamilton, Bermuda, March 9–14, 1975.
11. Jain, K. K., Some observations on the anatomy of the middle cerebral artery. Can. J. Surg. *7* (1964), 134–139.
12. Kaufman, B., The "empty" sella turcica – a manifestation of the intrasellar subarachnoid space. Radiology *90* (1968), 931–941.
13. Kaufman, B., Chamberlin, W. B., The ubiquitous sella turcica. Acta Radiol. *13* (1972), 413–425.
14. Kollmann, J., Lehrbuch der Entwicklungsgeschichte. Jena: G. Fischer. 1898.
15. Kollmannsberger, A., Vergleichende Studien über die A. Heubneri und die Aa. choroideae an anatomischen Präparaten, an Korrosionspräparaten und Angiogrammen der Hirngefäße. Morph. Jb. *102* (1961), 180–199.
16. Krayenbühl, H., Yaşargil, M. G., Die zerebrale Angiographie. Stuttgart: Thieme. 1965.
17. Lang, J., Clinical Anatomy of the Head. Neurocranium – Orbit – Craniocervical Regions. Berlin-Heidelberg-New York: Springer. 1983.
18. Lang, J., In: v. Lanz/Wachsmuth. Praktische Anatomie, übergeordnete Systeme. Part I, IA. Berlin-Heidelberg-New York: Springer. In print.
19. Lang, J., Brunner, F. K., Über die Rami centrales der Aa. cerebri anterior und media. Morph. Jb. *124* (1978), 364–374.
20. Lang, J., Häckel, H. R., Neue Befunde zum Verlauf der A. cerebri anterior (Pars postcommunicalis), zu den Abgangszonen und Weiten ihrer Rami corticales. Acta Anat. *108* (1980), 498–509.
21. Lang, J., Haas, R., Neue Befunde zur Bodenregion der Fossa cranialis anterior. Verh. Anat. Ges. *73* (1979), 77–86.
22. Lang, J., Schäfer, K., Über Ursprung und Versorgungsgebiete der intracavernösen Strecke der A. carotis interna. Morph. Jb. *122* (1976), 182–202.
23. McCormick, W. F., Vascular disorders of nervous tissue: Anomalies, malformations, and aneurysms. The structure and function of nervous tissue. In: Biochemistry and Disease, Vol. III, pp. 537–596. New York–London: Academic Press. 1969.
24. Mitterwallner, F. V., Variationsstatistische Untersuchungen an den basalen Hirngefäßen. Acta Anat. *24* (1955), 51–88.
25. Nomina Anatomica; 4th ed. (Approved by the 10th Int. Congr. of Anatomists, Tokyo 1975.) Amsterdam: Excerpta Medica. 1977.
26. Perlmutter, D., Rhoton, A. L., Microsurgical anatomy of the anterior cerebral–anterior communicating recurrent artery complex. J. Neurosurg. *45* (1976), 259–272.
27. Rahe, A. R., van der, Anomalous commissure of the 3rd ventricle (aberrant dorsal supraoptic decussation). A report on eight cases. Arch. Neurol. *37* (1937), 1283–1288.
28. Renn, W. H., Rhoton, A. L., Microsurgical anatomy of the sellar region. J. Neurosurg. *43* (1975), 288–298.
29. Riggs, H. E., Rupp, C., Variation in form of circle of Willis. Am. med. Ass. Arch. Neurol. *8* (1963), 24–30.
30. Robertson, G., The suprasellar region. In: Pneumoencephalography (Robertson, E. O., ed.), pp. 314–318. Springfield, Ill.: Ch. C Thomas. 1967.
31. Schmidt, H.-M., Über die postnatale Entwicklung der Vertikalabstände zwischen der Lamina cribrosa und kranimetrischen Meßpunkten und Schädelebenen. Verb. Anat. Ges. *69* (1975), 799–805.
32. Shealy, C. N., Jackson, C. C. R., Pearson, O., Kaufmann, B., Submucosal infranasal transphenoidal hypophysectomy. Bull. Los Angeles Neurol. Soc. *33* (1968), 185.
33. Spiegel, E. A., Wycis, H. T., Stereoencephalotomy (Thalamotomy and Related Procedures). New York: Grune & Stratton. 1952.

34. Stramrud, L., External and internal cranial base. A cross sectional study of growth and of association in form. Acta odont. Scand. *17* (1959), 239–266.

35. Tomasch, J., A quantitative analysis of the human anterior commissure. Acta anat. *30* (1957), 902–906.

36. Tomasch, J., The human posterior commissure. J. comp. Neurol. *124* (1965), 43–50.

37. Tseng, S.–L., Li, H., The external arteries of the brain in the Chinese (Chinese). Acta Anat. Sinica *8* (1965), 259–288.

38. Wollschlaeger, G., Wollschlaeger, P. B., Lucas, F. V., Lopez, V. F., Experience and result with postmortem cerebral angiography performed as routine procedure of the autopsy. Am. J. Roentgenol. *101* (1967), 68–87.

Author's address: Prof. Dr. med. Johannes Lang, Anatomisches Institut, Koellikerstrasse 6, D-8700 Würzburg, Federal Republic of Germany.

Acta Neurochirurgica, Suppl. 35, 23–30 (1985)

C. Pathology

Pathology of Midline Brain Tumors

Immunocytochemical Tumor Markers and Classificatory Aspects

H. Budka

Neurological Institute, University of Vienna, Wien, Austria

Summary

Our understanding of the pathology of human brain tumors has considerably increased in recent years thanks to investigation of nervous tissue markers which can be demonstrated by immunocytochemical techniques in sections of neurosurgical tissue specimens. This development is presented here in a review of the most important entities among midline brain tumors. Detection of neural differentiation markers such as glial fibrillary acidic protein (GFAP), S 100 protein (S 100 p), neurofibrillary proteins and neuron-specific enolase (NSE) greatly contributed to clarifying the histogenesis and differentiation potential of undifferentiated small-cell tumors grouped as primitive neuroectodermal tumors (PNETs) which include cerebellar medulloblastomas and pinealoblastomas as well as neuroblastomas and ependymoblastomas. Among medulloblastomas, the desmoplastic variety (formerly called by some "arachnoidal sarcoma of the cerebellum") shows frequent glioneuronal differentiation. Monoclonal antibodies recognizing antigenic determinants specific for tumor types and grades of malignancy/differentiation will gain significance in brain tumor diagnosis, as demonstrated in some examples. Despite the development of more objective ("scientific") criteria for typing human brain tumors, the "art" of classical histopathologic evaluation is not replaced but supplemented by the wealth of data supplied by such modern accomplishments.

Keywords: Brain tumor; glioma; tumor marker; immunocytochemistry; monoclonal antibodies; medulloblastoma; ependymoma; neurooncology.

1. Introduction

In recent years, remarkable progress has been made in our knowledge of the pathology of human brain tumors. Most of this progress resulted from investigations on a number of proteins ("markers") specific to the nervous system or playing an important role in nervous system function. Although there are so far only very few proteins which are exclusive for any one cell type, detection of nervous tissue markers is now routinely attempted in many neuropathological laboratories. Demonstration of neural cell markers in surgical tumor tissue specimens greatly contributes to increasing the diagnostic accuracy of histology [2], which still remains the basis of most prognostic and therapeutic considerations. Other recent approaches to increase the prognostic significance of neuropathological diagnosis include computerized multivariant analysis of a variety of histological features[10]. Such recent developments were designed to make the neuropathological tumor diagnosis less subjective, or—in other words—to shift it from the "art" of histopathology towards more objective ("scientific") criteria. It must be stressed, however, that diagnostic evaluation of tumor tissue still must rely on morphology, on the appropriate consideration of essentially unmeasurable criteria: Thus, the histopathologist's art is not likely to succumb soon to a dry compilation of physicochemical data.

It is beyond the scope of this presentation to give a fully comprehensive account of the pathology of midline brain tumors. Rather this is a very personal view of some recently emerging aspects of the classification of midline brain tumors and of those tumor markers which I consider clinically important.

2. Posterior Fossa Tumors

Traditionally, posterior fossa tumors are classified by their site as tumors of the cerebellum, brain stem, fourth ventricle and cerebellopontine angle. However, there is considerable overlap of these tumor locations. In many instances it is only a matter of academic interest if a neoplasm originated in the cerebellum and extended into the brainstem or *vice versa*; functional deficits remain the same for the patient. But there are clear-cut pathologic entities among posterior fossa tumors: primitive tumors including medulloblastomas, ependymomas, cerebellar astrocytomas, brain stem gliomas, neurilemomas (Schwannomas) and choroid plexus papillomas.

2.1. The Medulloblastoma and its Relation to Primitive Neuroectodermal Tumors (PNETs)

The embryonal nature of this common neoplasm of childhood is well recognized from the dense accumulation of small undifferentiated cellular elements. Routine histology and even electron microscopy usually fail to contribute much to the characterization of this tumor. However, the detection of differentiation markers (present in normal tissue and in differentiating neoplasms) by immunomorphological techniques revealed the capacity of medulloblastomas for divergent cellular differentiation. Immunocytochemical demonstration of neurofibrillary proteins and neuron specific enolase (NSE) (Fig. 1A) signal differentiation along neuronal lines, that of glial fibrillary acidic protein (GFAP) is evidence of astrocytic differentiation (Fig. 1B). In my experience, such signs of differentiation are mainly restricted to a peculiar subtype of medulloblastoma with a mosaic-like arrangement of less cellular islands amidst highly cellular streams with a high content of reticulin fibers. In this pure *desmoplastic variant*, both neuronal (Fig. 1 A) and glial (Fig. 1 B) differentiation markers are mainly expressed in the less cellular islands[14]. This differentiating capacity of the desmoplastic medulloblastoma is interesting with regard to reports that this variant carries a better

prognosis[8]. It is found more often in young adults and more frequently in a lateral site than the classical medulloblastoma. These characteristics are not undisputed[17], and also the better prognosis of the desmoplastic variant has been questioned[16, 17] when routine histological features have been considered. It remains to be seen if the identification of differentiation markers gains any prognostic significance.

Another exciting new development for better characterization of primitive tumors such as medulloblastomas is the possibility of labeling with monoclonal antibodies. These are powerful immunological reagents with homogeneity, defined specificity and physical properties. Usually a monoclonal antibody recognizes a small part of a molecule although a similar part of other molecules may also be recognized (cross-reactivity). When we recently tested a battery of monoclonal antibodies originally raised against hemopoietic cells, we found frequent cross-reactivities with brain tumors, in patterns characteristic for benign and/or malignant gliomas and/or PNETs[7]. Some of our antibodies are operationally specific within the nervous system and thus promise aid in neuropathological tumor diagnosis. An example for the diagnostic application of these monoclonal antibodies is given in Figs. 1 D–F: Intraopertively prepared smears from a cerebellar tumor of a 16-year-old male showed small regular cells separated by elongated cell forms in a routine cytological stain (Fig. 1C). Both medulloblastoma and cerebellar astrocytoma were considered, but a conclusion was not reached. Immunolabeling showed binding of an antibody, recognizing selectively glial cell processes, to some structures (Fig. 1E). Another antibody with specificity for PNETs labeled the tumor cell surfaces (Fig. 1F). Such a pattern of immunoreactivity suggested a diagnosis of PNET with some glial differentiation. Later histology confirmed this assumption; the diagnosis was desmoplastic medulloblastoma which is a PNET with frequent glial differentiation[14].

Fig. 1A and B. Desmoplastic medulloblastoma. Characteristic histological mosaic pattern of fiber- and cell-rich tissue surrounding slightly less cellular islands without reticulin fibers. Immunocytochemistry reveals diffuse expression of neuron-specific enolase (NSE) within the islands (dark reaction product in A); glial differentiation signaled by immunolabeling of glial fibrillary acidic protein (GFAP) is mainly restricted to the islands (B). C Cytological evidence of postoperative CSF seeding of medulloblastoma. A densely cellular tumor aggregate is found in the lumbar CSF 5 days after operation for medulloblastoma. D–F Intraoperative smear preparations of a cerebellar tumor in a 16-year-old male. Routine cytological stain (D) shows small regular cells separated by elongated cell forms-cerebellar astrocytoma or medulloblastoma? Immunolabeling shows binding of monoclonal antibody VIT 13 to moderately many cell processes (E) and of antibody VIB C5 to all cell membranes (F). VIT 13 is an antibody labeling glial cell processes, VIB C5 labels all primitive neuroectodermal tumors (PNET). The pattern of immunoreactivity of this tumor suggested a diagnosis of PNET with some glial differentiation. Later histology confirmed this assumption with the diagnosis of desmoplastic medulloblastoma which is a PNET with frequent differentiation (cf., Figs. 1 A, B). A and B peroxidase-antiperoxidase technique on paraffin sections, A × 250, Nomarski optics; B × 150, slight nuclear counterstain. C May-Grünwald-Giemsa stain of CSF sediment, × 250, Nomarski optics. D–F smears from fresh tissue; D May-Grünwald-Giemsa, × 630; E and F indirect immunofluorescent technique, E × 250, F × 160

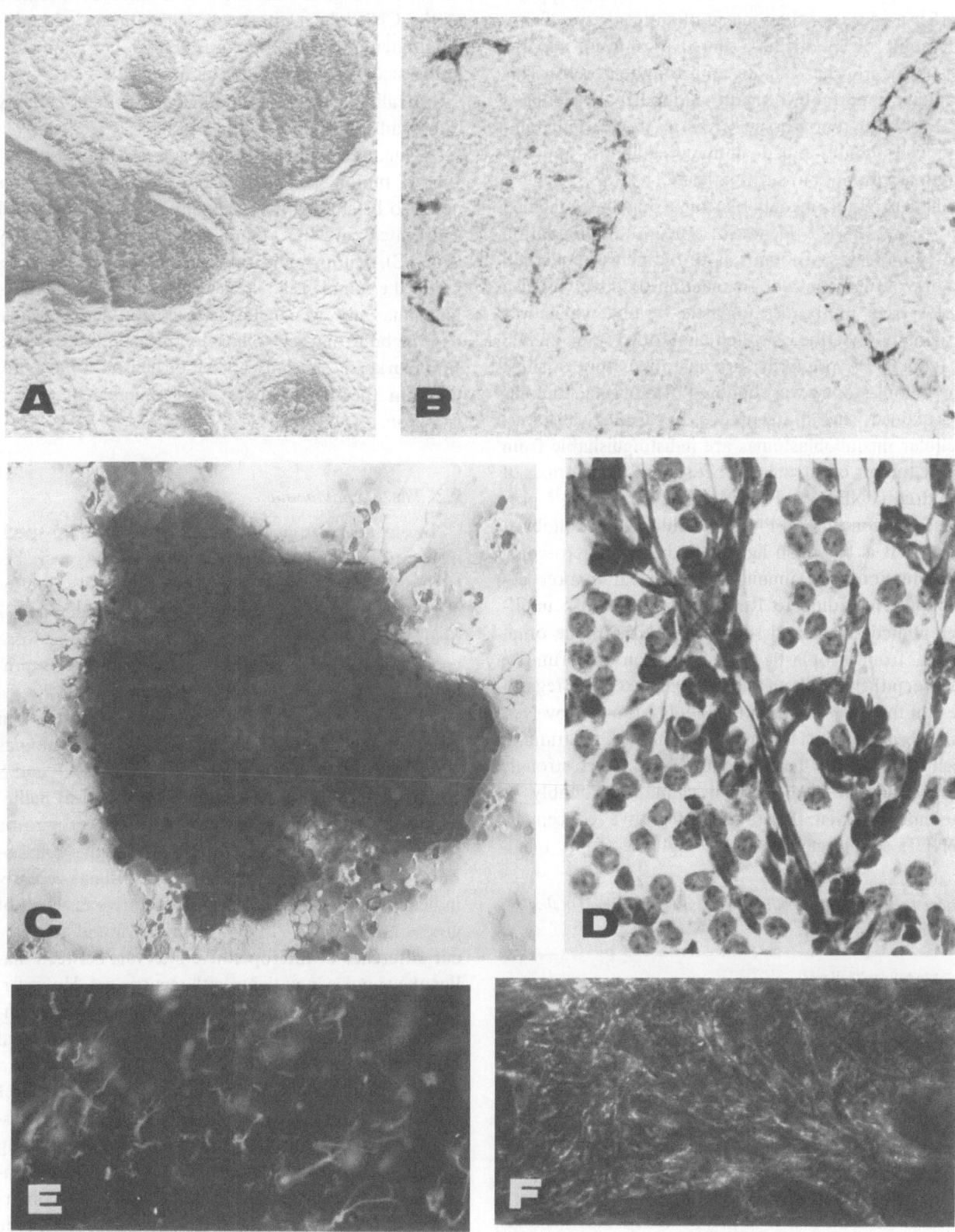

Fig. 1

Our study with monoclonal antibodies also supports earlier evidence of the concept of antigenic specificity, or family of specificities, shared by normal nervous tissue, neurogenic tumors and lymphoid cells. This could be important when auto-antibodies are produced against brain tumor tissue: Cross-reaction with lymphoid cells could impair immunoregulation and the immune response in such patients[6].

The origin of medulloblastomas has been debated for decades. The evidence for a neural differentiation potential leaves no doubt as to the neuroectodermal nature of this neoplasm. As mentioned above, this also holds true for the desmoplastic variant, which was originally described as "circumscribed arachnoidal sarcoma"[9]. A primarily sarcomatous nature of most medulloblastomas was supposed by Gullotta[12] but has not gained general acceptance. In histological terms, cellular medulloblastomas are indistinguishable from some tumors occurring at other sites of the neuraxis of children (PNETs[13]). Resently, Lucy B. Rorke[18] proposed a concept of PNETs including medulloblastomas: It is based on light and electron microscopic examinations and immunocytochemical marker detection. According to Rorke[18], the cell-dense undifferentiated small- and round-cell PNET tissue originates from neoplastic transformation of primitive neuroepithelial cells of subependymal regions regardless of the site. Cerebellar medulloblastomas, however, have been reported to originate from the fetal granular cell layer[19]. The term medulloblastoma is strongly entrenched in medicine[23]; it cannot reasonably be abandoned even if Rorke's integrative concept of PNETs should gain general acceptance. Table 1 outlines a histological classification of embryonal tumors of the CNS which appreciates the concept of undifferentiated or differentiating PNETs[18], but retains the terms medulloblastoma and desmoplastic[5].

Medulloblastomas are notorious for their capacity to spread along CSF pathways. This is frequently a spontaneous event. However, the possibilitiy of dispersion of tumor elements during operative procedures needs to be studied. Occasionally, I found tumor cell aggregates in the lumbar CSF postoperatively (Fig. 1C). Autopsy confirmed later extensive CSF seeding of the tumor. Like other types of PNET, medulloblastomas may even metastasize to extraneural organs, e.g. the bone marrow. Detection of neural differentiation markers, especially GFAP or neurofibrillary proteins, in the metastasis is most valuable in such a situation.

2.2. The Ependymoma

In our neurosurgical tissue material of 9,705 specimens submitted for neuropathological diagnosis between 1964 and 1984 (vertebral disc tissue not included), a diagnosis of ependymoma was made in 177 operations (1.8%) on 131 patients. Posterior fossa ependymomas were slightly less frequent than supratentorial ones (33% vs. 40% of operations; 35% vs. 37% of patients; 27% of ependymoma operations in 28% of patients were spinal). Many ependymomas express the glial differentiation markers GFAP and S 100 protein (S 100 p). Grading of histological malignancy does not seem to have as much prognostic significance as in astroglial tumors, although a collaborative study on supratentorial ependymomas recently indicated some differences in postoperative survivals of grades I, II, and III[1]. In our material, I found no clear-cut difference of interoperative intervals between malignancy grades in patients with recurrences. However, it was interesting to note that one third of all recurrences had a higher malignancy grade than the original tumor. Posterior fossa ependymomas usually have a uniform benign appearance corresponding to grade I (79%, including the histological subtype of "subependymoma", a variant with a frequently dominating fibrillary astroglial component). In contrast, supratentorial ependymomas tend to be much more pleomorphic: Only 33% were graded as I, but 36% were grade III and 31% grade II. As suggested by Collin's law, age seems to have some prognostic influence. In 31 patients with intracranial recurring ependymoma the interval until recurrence was 12.37 ± 6.44 months in infants (0–

Table 1. *Histological Classification of Embryonal Tumors of the CNS* (Budka 1984)

1. Medulloepithelioma
2. *Primitive neuroectodermal tumor* (PNET) including
   Medulloblastoma (cerebellar PNET) and
   Pinealoblastoma (pineal PNET)

   Supplementary designation: *desmoplastic* (to be added in tumors with a prominent mesenchymal component)

   Subgroups: a. *without differentiation*
               b. *with differentiation*
   i. glial (astrocytic and/or oligodendroglial)
   ii. ependymal (ependymoblastoma)
   iii. neuronal (also neuroblastoma and ganglioneuroblastoma)
   iv. bi- or pluripotential

3. Medullomyoblastoma
4. Primitive polar spongioblastoma
5. Others

4 years), 18.6 ± 18.16 in children (age 6–15) and 14.66 ± 10.38 in adults (older than 20). However, overall prognosis seems grim for all ages even in tumors with benign histological features[21]. More or less differentiated ependymomatous areas may accompany otherwise cell-dense primitive tumors, defining a special variant of differentiating PNETs, the ependymoblastoma (Table 1). This latter entity, usually restricted to infants and children, must not be confused with anaplastic (grade III) ependymomas preferring older age.

2.3. The Choroid Plexus Papilloma

This relatively rare tumor has a characteristic benign papillary histology. Its malignant variant ("choroid plexus carcinoma") is very rare and usually occurs in infancy. In my experience, some of these malignant tumors contain solid small-cell parts indistinguishable from PNETs, in addition to more classical choroidal papillae; also, areas reminiscent of ependymoma or ependymoblastoma may be found. *Primitive papillary tumors of infancy* would be the appropriate designation for such a complex histological picture.

Histological differential diagnosis of papillary brain tumors in older age is very difficult since metastases of papillary adeno-carcinoma must be considered in addition to choroid plexus papilloma and papillary ependymoma. In my experience, a set of three markers is most helpful for clinching the differential diagnosis. Secretory component, the protein linking secretory immunoglobulins in normal and neoplastic secretory epithelium, is demonstrable by immunohistology in metastatic adenocarcinoma, but absent in primary papillary brain tumors. I found this immunocytochemical pattern in 20 metastases and 10 primary tumors. Furthermore, metastatic carcinoma lacks immunocytochemical expression of S 100 p. GFAP and S 100 p are also useful for distinguishing between choroid plexus papilloma (strongly positive for S 100 p, but negative or only focally positive for GFAP) and papillary ependymoma (usually positive for both markers[15]).

2.4. Cerebellar Astrocytoma and Brainstem Glioma

These tumors are the most common infratentorial tumors of childhood. Despite their common astroglial histogenesis, they differ greatly in behaviour and prognosis. Cerebellar astrocytoma of childhood and adolescence usually is represented by the histological variant of *pilocytic astrocytoma,* named after the elongated shape of many constituting cells. It is most important to recognize this variety in histological reports and statistics, since it can be regarded as the most benign of all gliomas. Cure or at least remission for decades is achieved by resection, and malignant evolution is extremely rare[3]. Brainstem glioma by contrast, usually does not belong to the true pilocytic astrocytoma type, although its tumor cells may align alongside nerve fiber tracts in an elongated ("pseudo-pilocytic") cell shape. The main characteristic of this tumor is its diffuse, non-delineated growth usually respecting much of the preexisting nervous parenchyma but frequently condensing in anaplastic foci with central necrosis (Fig. 2A). When I studied large-sized histological sections of brainstem gliomas at autopsy, all 12 tumors had at least one anaplastic focus despite of benign-looking features elsewhere.

3. Supratentorial Tumors

Supratentorial tumors of the midline in infancy and childhood usually comprise less malignant tumor types than the lateral regions[11]. This is especially true for tumors of hypothalamus, optic nerve, third ventricle and foramen of Monro regions, but less so for neoplasms of the pineal region. Some malignant tumors may extend via the skull base to the intracranial cavity and present as basal midline masses, e.g. lymphomas or sarcomas, especially embryonal rhabdomyosarcomas (Fig. 2B) originating from the orbit or middle ear.

3.1. Pineal Tumors

A classification of the major groups of pineal neoplasms is given in Table 2. Tumors arising from specific pineal parenchymal cells, the true pinealomas, constitute only a minority. The pinealoblastoma usually is indistinguishable from the undifferentiated pattern of PNETs (Table 1), but may infrequently show tubular rosettes similar to retinoblastomas or signs of glioneuronal differentiation[20]. Such tumors may widely

Table 2. *Classification of Pineal Tumors (Major Groups)*

1. Germ cell tumors
2. True pinealomas
   a. Pinealocytoma
   b. Pinealoblastoma
3. Gliomas
4. Pineal cysts
5. Others

extend anteriorly or into the posterior fossa. It may become impossible to differentiate a posteriorly growing pinealoblastoma from an anteriorly extending cerebellar medulloblastoma. Germ cell tumors are the most common tumors of the pineal region. They do not differ in morphology or behaviour from their counterparts in the gonads, and must be classified accordingly. Since germ cell tumors may have only very small parts of a component which may be decisive for prognosis and appropriate therapy, it is important to submit as much of the tumor as possible to painstaking histological analysis. Small sterotactic biopsies may not reveal the full scope of the tumor. On thorough search, even teratomas (by many regarded as very benign lesions) reveal malignant components in a very high proportion of cases[4].

Gliomas of the pineal region (Fig. 2C) may be difficult to differentiate from neighbouring cerebral tumors extending to the pineal region. However, the behaviour of parapineal and pineal gliomas does not seem to differ.

3.2. Hypothalamic Tumors

Among non-neural tumors, suprasellar extension of pituitary adenomas usually are well-delineated, frequently by a fibrous capsule. By contrast craniopharyngiomas usually show strong tendencies to invade the hypothalamus, initiating vigorous fibrillary gliosis which may be mistaken by the histopathologist, in the absence of epithelial structures diagnostic of craniopharyngioma, as astroglial neoplasm. Very large craniopharyngiomas may extend through the third ventricle to the corpus callosum (Fig. 2F).

Hypothalamic germ cell tumors do not behave differently from their pineal counterparts. They tend to seed along CSF pathways and may ensheath much of the spinal cord and roots (Fig. 2E).

Among true parenchymal tumors of the hypothalamus, the hypothalamic hamartoma is a nodule abutting on the floor of the third ventricle, composed of regularly ordered neurons. This lesion usually lacks signs of expansion, respects other anatomical structures (Fig. 2D) and is more similar to a malformation than to a true neoplasm. The most common hypothalamic tumor is pilocytic astrocytoma, comparable to cerebellar astrocytoma. These histologically benign tumors may be of giant size, replacing and compressing much of the basal structures. Even vessels may be displaced and compressed to such an extent that infarction may occur (Fig. 2G).

3.3. Optic (Nerve) Gliomas

Although malignant tumors may rarely arise in the anterior optic pathways, the common optic nerve glioma is a very benign neoplasm with a tendency to invade the optic sheaths. Despite the usual lack of sharp delineation and development of cysts, other characteristics of this tumor correspond to pilocytic astrocytomas in other sites.

3.4. Tumors of the Foramen of Monro Region

A wide variety of lesions may block the CSF pathways at the foramen of Monro. Two entities, however, usually do not present elsewhere in the brain. The *colloid cyst* (of the third ventricle), despite its characteristic appearance and location, may have more than one origin. Many colloid cysts have a lining indistinguishable by morphological criteria from ependyma; others may contain mucous goblet cells and even squamous epithelium supporting a non-neuroepithelial origin[22].

The *subependymal giant cell astrocytoma usually* occurs as a ventricle tumor of the tuberous sclerosis complex. Despite the bizarre appearance of its cells, it is generally a lesion with benign behaviour. Since tuberous sclerosis affects the whole neuraxis, symptoms may be due not only to CSF blocking by the foramen of Monro tumor, but also to accompanying lesions elsewhere in the brain (Fig. 2H). In my experience this

---

Fig. 2. *A* Brainstem glioma causing enormous swelling of pons; however, architecture of myelinated fiber tracts (dark) and nuclei is largely preserved. An anaplastic tumor focus stands out by necrosis (n). *B* An infantile skull base tumor presenting as basal midline lesion; occasional cross-striation (arrowhead) identifies this primitive tumor tissue as embryonal rhabdomyosarcoma. *C* Anaplastic astrocytoma of the pineal region. *D* Hypothalamic hamartoma; normal anatomical structures including mamillary bodies are intact. *E* CSF seeding in a malignant germ cell tumor originating from the hypothalamus; large tumor plate on the dorsal surface of the spinal cord. *F* Giant-sized craniopharyngioma extends from the flattened sella through the third ventricle to the callosal splenium. Large cysts and gritty calcifications of the tumor are well seen on this median-sagittal section of brain and skull base. *G* Large pilocytic astrocytoma of hypothalamic region. The well-delineated tumor had compressed the basal arteries mainly on the right side, causing an old infarction in the right hemisphere. *H* Tuberous sclerosis. A subependymal giant cell astrocytoma blocks the foramen of Monro region more on the right side, with ensuing ventricular dilatation. There are also small subependymal tumor foci (arrowheads) and many cortical tubers (arrows). *A, D, G* and *H* luxol fast blue stain for myelin, counterstain with nuclear fast red. *B* PTAH stain, *E H, E* stain. Magnification: $A \times 1$; $B \times 630$; $D \times 1.7$; $E \times 3$; G and $H \times 0.5$

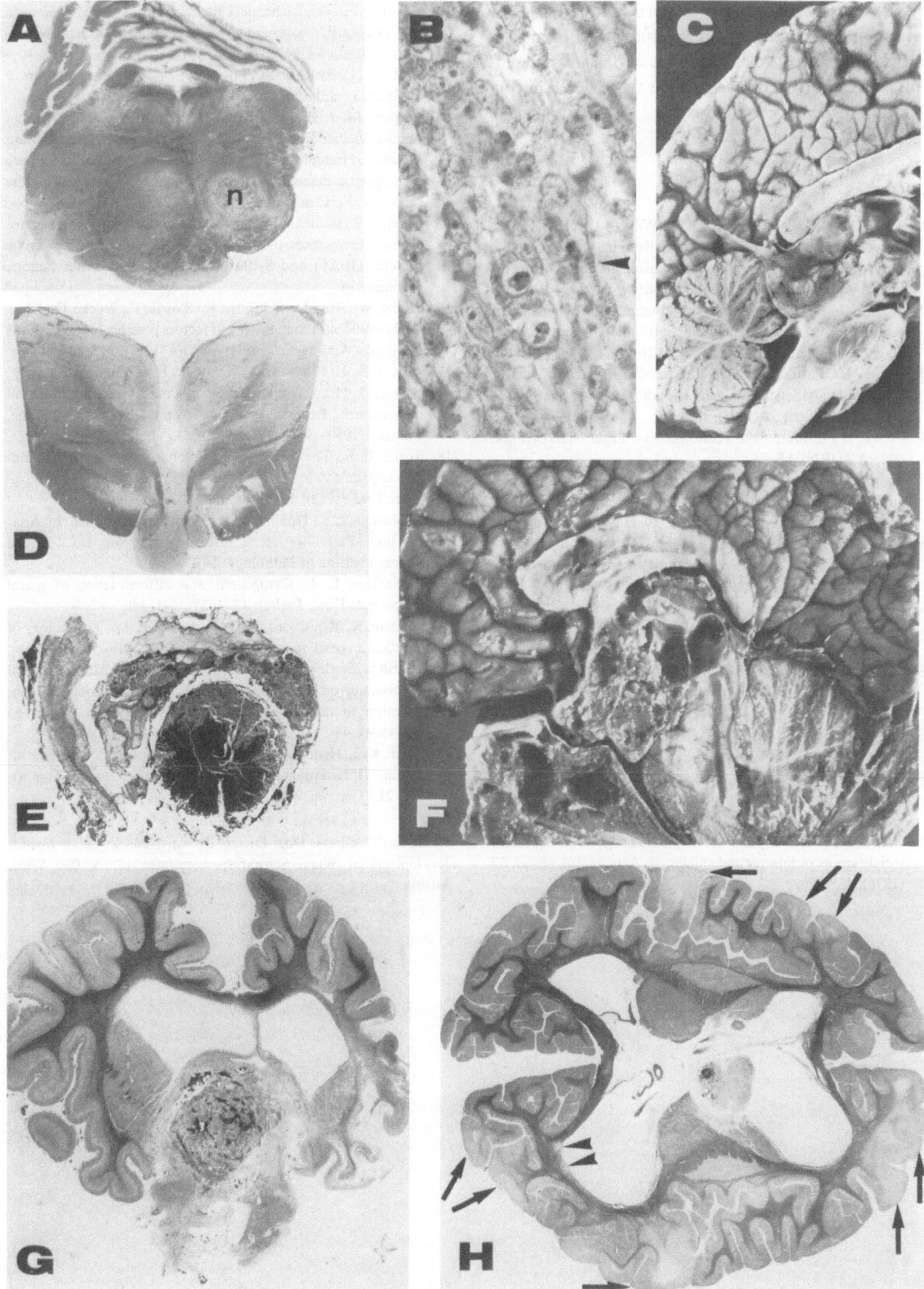

Fig. 2

tumor shows an outstanding pattern of immunoreactivity for neural markers; GFAP and S 100 p may be surprisingly scarce, whereas NSE is strongly expressed. This suggests origin from a peculiar type of cell sharing glial and neuronal characteristics.

References

1. Afra, D., Müller, W., Slowik, F., Wilcke, O., Budka, H., Turoczy, L., Supratentorial lobar ependymomas: Reports on the grading and survival periods in 80 cases, including 46 recurrences. Acta Neurochir. (Wien) *69* (1983), 243–251.
2. Bonnin, J. M., Rubinstein, L. J., Immunohistochemistry of central nervous system tumors. Its contribution to neurosurgical diagnosis. J. Neurosurg. *60* (1984), 1121–1133.
3. Budka, H., Partially resected and irradiated cerebellar astrocytoma of childhood: Malignant evolution after 28 years. Acta Neurochir. (Wien) *32* (1975), 129–146.
4. Budka, H., Intrakranielle Teratome. Akt. Probl. Neuropathol. (Wien) *2* (1978), 88–93.
5. Budka, H., Tumoren des Zentralnervensystems. In: Histologische Tumorklassifikation (Österr. Ges. Pathol., Hrsg.) pp. 140–146. Wien-New York: Springer. 1984.
6. Budka, H., Majdic, O., Shared antigenic determinants between human hemopoietic cells and nervous tissues and tumors. Acta Neuropathol. (Berl.) *67* (1985), 58–66.
7. Budka, H., Majdic, O., Knapp, W., Cross-reactivity between human hemopoietic cells and brain tumors as defined by monoclonal antibodies. J. Neuro-Oncol. *3* (1985), 173–179.
8. Chatty, E. M., Earle, K. M., Medulloblastoma. A report of 201 cases with emphasis on the relationship of histologic variants to survival. Cancer *28* (1971), 977–983.
9. Förster, O., Gagel, O., Das umschriebene Arachnoidalsarkom des Kleinhirns. Z. Ges. Neurol. Psychiat. *164* (1938), 565–580.
10. Gilles, F. H., Leviton, A., Hedley-Whyte, E. T., Jasnow, M., Childhood brain tumor update. Hum. Pathol. *14* (1983), 834–845.
11. Gjerris, F., Clinical aspects and long-term prognosis in supratentorial tumors of infancy and childhood. Acta neurol. scand. *57* (1978), 445–470.
12. Gullotta, F., Vergleichende Untersuchungen zur Morphologie und Genese der sogenannten Medulloblastome. Acta Neuropathol. (Berl.) *8* (1967), 76–83.
13. Hart, M. N., Earle, K. M., Primitive neuroectodermal tumors of the brain in children. Cancer *32* (1973), 890–897.
14. Herpers, M. J. H. M., Budka, H., Primitive neuroectodermal tumors including the medulloblastoma: glial differentiation signaled by immunoreactivity for GFAP is restricted to the pure desmoplastic medulloblastoma ("arachnoidal sarcoma of the cerebellum"). Clin. Neuropathol. *4* (1985), 12–18.
15. Kimura, T., Budka, H., Soler-Federsppiel, F., An immunocytochemical comparison of the glia cell markers glial fibrillary acidic protein (GFAP) and S-100 protein in human brain tumors. (Submitted.)
16. Müller, W., Afra, D., Schröder, R., Slowik, F., Wilcke, O., Klug, N., Medulloblastoma: Survey of factors possibly influencing the prognosis. Acta Neurochir. (Wien) *64* (1982), 215–224.
17. Park, T. S., Hoffman, H. J., Hendrick, E. B., Humphreys, R. P., Becker, L. E., Medulloblastoma: Clinical presentation and management. Experience at the Hospital For Sick Children, Toronto, 1950–1980. J. Neurosurg. *58* (1983), 543–552.
18. Rorke, L. B., The cerebellar medulloblastoma and its relationship to primitive neuroectodermal tumors. J. Neuropathol. Exp. Neurol. *42* (1983), 1–15.
19. Rubinstein, L. J., Tumors of the central nervous system. In: Atlas of Tumor Pathology, ser. 2, fasc. 6. Washington, D.C.: Armed Forces Institute of Pathology. 1972.
20. Rubinstein, L. J., Cytogenesis and differentiation of pineal neoplasms. Hum. Pathol. *12* (1981), 441–448.
21. Shuman, R. M., Alvord, E. C., jr., Leech, R. W., The biology of childhood ependymomas. Arch. Neurol. *32* (1975), 731–739.
22. Yagishita, S., Itoh, Y., Shiozawa, T., Tanaka, T., Ultrastructural observation on a colloid cyst of the third ventricle. A contribution to its pathogenesis. Acta Neuropathol. (Berl.) *65* (1984), 41–45.
23. Zülch, K. J., Histological typing of tumors of the central nervous system. (International Histological Classification of Tumors, No. 21.) Geneva: WHO. 1979.

Author's address: Doz. Dr. H. Budka, Neurologisches Institut der Universität Wien, Schwarzspanierstrasse 17, A-1090 Wien, Austria.

Acta Neurochirurgica, Suppl. 35, 31–41 (1985)

D. Approaches

Problems of Surgical Technique for the Treatment of Supratentorial Midline Tumors in Children

W. T. Koos, A. Perneczky, and **A. Horaczek**

Department of Neurosurgery, University of Vienna Medical School, Wien, Austria

Summary

In this presentation the authors describe briefly their thoughts on microsurgical management of certain typical brain tumors arising from within and adjacent to the third ventricle the surgical treatment of which has for many years been essentially conservative, not infrequently without histological verification of the type of the tumor or even of the presence of a real neoplasm.

Keywords: Brain tumors in children; cerebral midline; surgical approaches; microneurosurgical techniques.

Introduction

Tumors of the supratentorial midline region, particularly those of the third ventricle, comprise an interesting group of lesions which have intrigued neurosurgeons for decades because of their difficult accessibility[8, 12, 35, 39–43, 73, 80].

The third ventricle and the paraventricular areas harbor an unusually wide variety of pathological processes (Fig. 1)[31, 100].

Surgical Considerations

The selection of the best operative approach for a diagnosed tumor of the third ventricle depends on the site of origin, direction of growth, and location of the tumor in relation to the various sections of the ventricle, the site of compression of the ventricle, and whether there is ventricular obstruction with corresponding hydrocephalus.

When discussing surgery of third ventricular tumors, it is important to consider the proportions of tumor that are encapsulated, have discrete areas of attachment, and are presumably resectable if an appropriate approach can be used. In approximately 40% of the lesions, an optimum situation exists so that surgical resection may be accomplished. In the remaining instances little more than partial resection or biopsy of the neoplasm can be done without significantly jeopardizing the patient. A guiding principle of any surgical approach must be that the removal of neural tissue and sacrifice of anatomical structures should be minimized. The former high mortality of third ventricle tumor surgery, which prompted a more conservative approach, has been significantly decreased by the use of the operating microscope and of highly sophisticated microsurgical techniques. Reports of total removal of benign tumors with excellent results are being reported everywhere[8, 57, 75, 76, 78, 82, 87, 90, 94, 97].

A survey of standard approaches to supratentorial midline tumors are shown in Fig. 2 and listed in Table 1.

Schematic depictions of the various approaches to intra- and paraventricular lesions (as listed in Fig. 2) are presented in detail in Figs. 3 to 14.

TUMORS OF THE THIRD VENTRICLE

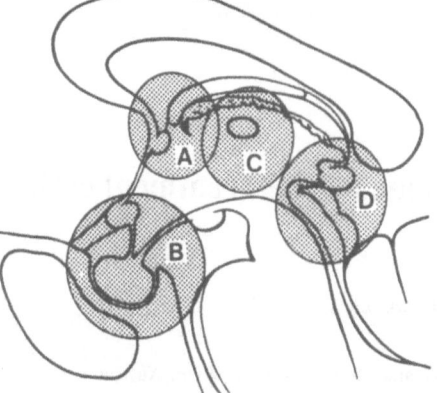

A: ANTERIOR (ORAL) GROUP

  INTRAVENTRICULAR:

    EPENDYMAL (COLLOID) CYSTS
    CHOROID PLEXUS PAPILLOMAS
    EPIDERMOIDS
    (MENINGIOMAS)

  PARAVENTRICULAR:

    GLIOMAS OF SEPTUM PELLUCIDUM:

      ASTROCYTOMAS
      SPONGIOBLASTOMAS
      EPENDYMOMAS

      (MENINGIOMAS OF VELUM
       INTERPOSITUM)

B: INFERIOR (BASAL) GROUP

  PRIMARY INTRAVENTRICULAR:

    ASTROCYTOMAS (SPONGIOBLASTOMAS)
    CRANIOPHARYNGIOMAS
    GANGLIOCYTOMAS

  SECONDARY INTRAVENTRICULAR:

    (IMPLANTATION METASTASES)
    "ECTOPIC" PINEALOMAS
    MEDULLOBLASTOMAS

  PARAVENTRICULAR:

    CRANIOPHARYNGIOMAS
    (PITUITARY ADENOMAS)
    (MENINGIOMAS)
    (EPIDERMOIDS/DERMOIDS)

C: LATERAL GROUP

  PARAVENTRICULAR:

    ASTROCYTOMAS
    GLIOBLASTOMAS
    OLIGODENDROGLIOMAS

D: POSTERIOR (CAUDAL) GROUP

  INTRAVENTRICULAR:

    PINEOBLASTOMAS
    (MEDULLOBLASTOMAS)
    EPENDYMOMAS
    TERATOMAS
    PINEALOMAS
    EPENDYMAL CYSTS

  PARAVENTRICULAR:

    GLIOMAS (QUADRIGEMINAL PLATE)

      GLIOBLASTOMAS
      SPONGIOBLASTOMAS

    (MENINGIOMAS)

Fig. 1. Regional distribution of surgically accessible supratentorial midline brain tumors within and adjacent to the third ventricle according to their histological appearance (tumor types)

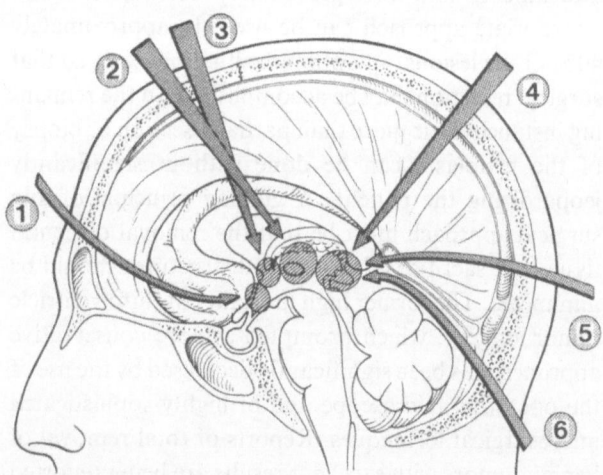

Fig. 2. Schematic presentation of the various approaches to supratentorial midline tumors: *1* Anterior basal approaches; *2* Interhemispheric transcallosal approaches; *3* Transfrontal transcortical transventricular approaches; *4* Parietal (posterior) interhemispheric transcallosal approach and transparietal transcortical transventricular approach; *5* Occipital transtentorial approach; *6* Infratentorial supracerebellar approach

Post-operative Complications

Post-operative Hydrocephalus

Even after successful removal of benign intraventricular tumors such as colloid cysts, etc., precautions must be taken with regard to post-operative hydrocephalus. Aqueductal stenosis or even occlusion may result from intra-operative drainage of the liquid contents of intraventricular cysts into the cerebrospinal fluid causing aseptic ependymitis. To prevent this complication the patient should be kept on ventricular drainage following surgery. Post-operative hydrocephalus or increase of a pre-operative hydrocephalus occurred in more than 20% of all supratentorial midline operations.

Cerebral Hemisphere Collaps

This complication may follow the decompression of a grossly enlarged ventricular system, particularly in children. Even though the hydrocephalic lateral ventricle facilitates exposure of the tumor, it is considered

Table 1. *Surgical Approaches to Supratentorial Midline Lesions*

Methods of approach	Approached regions and anatomical structures
Anterior basal approaches (Figs. 3, 4, and 5)	*Sella turcica—optic chiasm region, anterior and inferior portions of third ventricle.*

Unilateral subfrontal (Figs. 4/*1 a* and 5)
    transsphenoidal (Fig. 5/*1a*)
    pre- or subchiasmatic (Fig. 5/*1b*)
    retrochiasmatic or lamina terminals (Fig. 5/2)
    optico-carotid (Fig. 5/3)
	Both optic nerves and optic chasm, space between ipsilateral optic nerve and internal carotid artery, medial aspect of contralateral internal carotid artery, medial aspect of contralateral internal carotid artery, prechiasmatic region in case of pre-fixed chiasm, suprasellar region, lamina terminalis in case of prefixed chiasm.

Bilateral subfrontal
    transsphenoidal (Fig. 5/*1a*)
    pre- or subchiasmatic (Fig. 5/*1b*)
    retrochiasmatic or lamina terminals (Fig. 5/2)
	Both optic nerves and optic chiasm, prechiasmatic region in case of pre fixed chiasm, suprasellar region in case of postfixed chiasm, infundibulum, internal carotid arteries, retrochiasmatic region and lamina terminals in case of prefixed chiasm, anterior and inferior third ventricle.

Frontolateral (Figs. 4/*1b* and 5/3) optico-carotid (Fig. 5/3)	Ipsilateral optic nerve and optic tract, contralateral optic nerve internal carotid arteries, optic chiasm, suprasellar region, supra- and retrochiasmatic region (prefixed chiasm), space between ipsilateral optic nerve and internal carotid artery, parasellar region.
Pterional (Figs. 4/*1c* and 5/4)	Same as "frontolateral", in addition: Space between internal carotid artery and oculomotor nerve, subchiasmatic region, parasellar region hypothalamic area—infundibulum, retrosellar region, anterior "tentorial notch".
Frontotemporal and subtemporal (Fig. 5/5)	Same as "pterional", in addition: Ipsilateral part of arterial circle of Willis, subchiasmatic region, infundibulum, hypothalamic region, parasellar regionn, retrosellar region, tentorial notch, interpeduncular cistern, upper section of basilar artery, anterior and lateral aspect of midbrain, inferior portion of third ventricle.
Transcortical approaches (Fig. 7)	(Optimal in case of enlarged lateral ventricles) *Lateral ventricles, third ventricle.*
Transfrontal (Fig. 7)	Ipsilateral lateral ventricle.

Transfrontal transventricular
    transforaminal (Fig. 7/*1*)
    transseptal (Fig. 7/2)
    transfornical (Fig. 9/*A*)
    subchorioidal or interthalamus-trigonalis (Fig. 9/*B*)
	Ipsilateral foramen of Monro.
	Anterior third ventricle
	Controlateral lateral ventricle, contralateral foramen of Monro.
	Anterior and inferior part of third ventricle.
	Middle and anterior-superior portion of third ventricle.

Transparietal transventricular (Fig. 10)
    (parieto-temporal)
    parietal
	Trigone and posterior part of ipsilateral lateral ventricle, glomus of choroid plexus, pineal region.

Midline transcallosal approaches (Figs. 11 and 12)	(Lateral ventricles of normal size or minimally enlarged) *Lateral ventricles, entire third ventricle, pineal and quadrigeminal region.*
Interhemispheric transcallosal (uni- and/or bilateral, medial) anterior transcallosal (Figs. 11 and 12)	Ipsilateral and /or contralateral lateral ventricles. Anterior horns and cella media of both lateral ventricles, both foramina of Monro, anterior and superior part of third ventricle.

transforaminal
        transseptal
        transfornical
        subchoroidal or interthalamus-trigonalis
        interfornical
    posterior transcallosal (Fig. 11)
	(see "transcortical approaches")
	(see "transcortical approaches")
	(see "transcortical approaches")
	(see "transcortical approaches")
	Entire third ventricle, particularly superior, anterior and middle parts.
	Posterior (caudal) part of third ventricle, posterior part of corpus callosum, pineal and quadrigeminal plate region.

Posterior approaches (Fig. 14)	*Posterior third ventricle, pineal and quadrigeminal plate region, midbrain.*
Occipital transtentorial (Fig. 14)	Pineal and quadrigeminal plate region, posterior third ventricle.
Infratentorial supracerebellar (Fig. 14)	Pineal and quadrigeminal plate region, posterior third ventricle, midbrain, upper cerebellar midline.

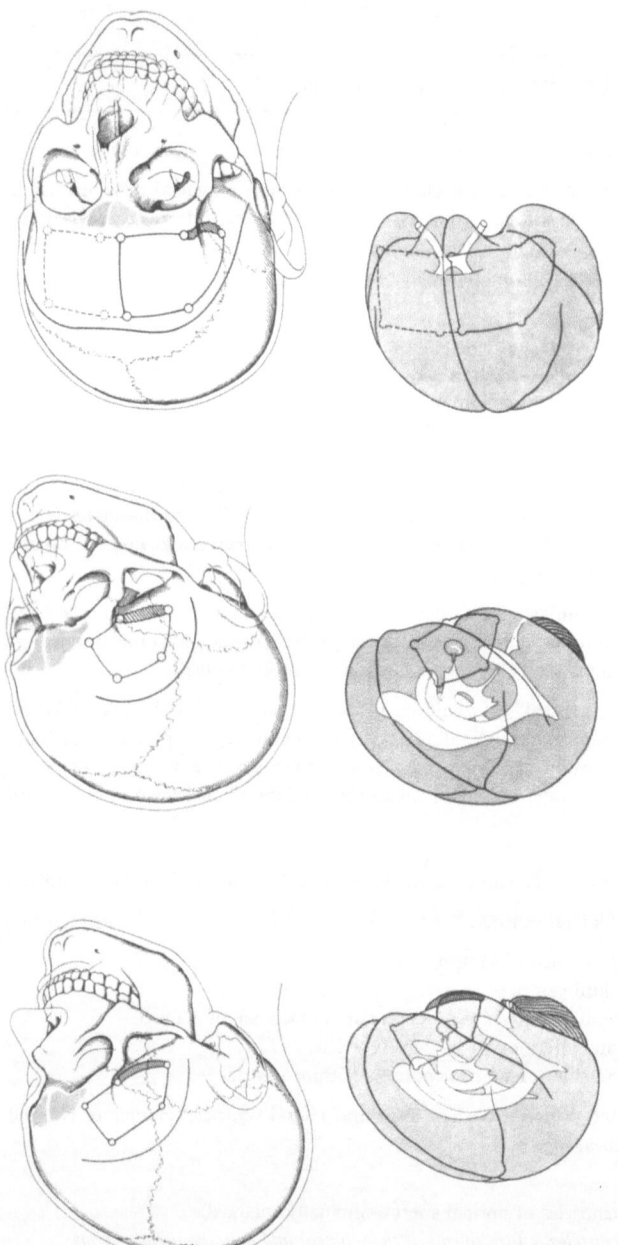

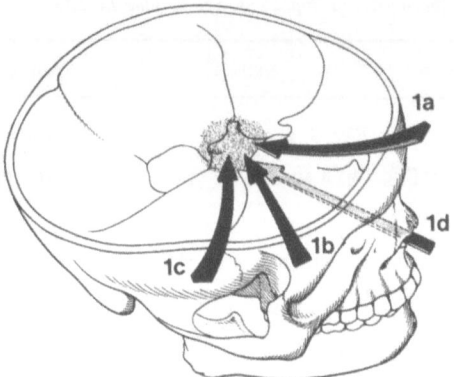

Fig. 4. The arrows depict the various approaches to the sellar, supra- and parasellar regions: *1a* subfrontal approach; *1b* frontolateral approach; *1c* pterional approach; *1d* transnasal-transphenoidal approach

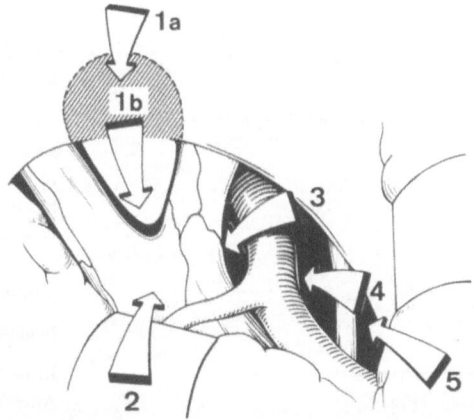

Fig. 5. Overview of the various anterior basal approaches (see Table 1): *1a* subfrontal transphenoidal approach (prefixed chiasm!); *1b* subfrontal prechiasmatic or subchiasmatic approach (postfixed chiasm!); *2* subfrontal retrochiasmatic or lamina terminalis-approach (prefixed chiasm!); *3* frontolateral approach; *4* pterional approach; *5* frontotemporal and subtemporal approach

Fig. 3. Schematic presentation of the various anterior basal approaches: Unilateral or bilateral subfrontal approach (above), frontolateral approach (middle), and pterional approach (below). The various scalp incisions are outlined and the relationship between the craniotomy, the cerebral hemispheres, the ventricular system and the underlying neural structures is demonstrated.

Problems Related to the Division of the Corpus Callosum[2, 3, 4, 8, 15, 34, 42, 52, 56, 73, 80, 81, 84, 85, 88]

Division of a modest portion of the anterior corpus callosum in our experience has not resulted in neurological deficits, provided the anterior cerebral arteries are kept intact. A longitudinal incision of the central or middle part of the corpus callosum may cause impairments related to the interhemispheric transfer of information and may result in significant learning problems in younger children. Additional laceration or interruption of the anterior commissure will cause severe memory problems. Furthermore, it is generally accepted that section of the posterior corpus callosum for extirpating thalamic and large pineal tumors will

expediant to relieve the hydrocephalus gradually by a shunting procedure to one or both lateral ventricles prior to a direct attack upon the tumor. If subdural hygroma becomes a problem, the subdural space may also be shunted.

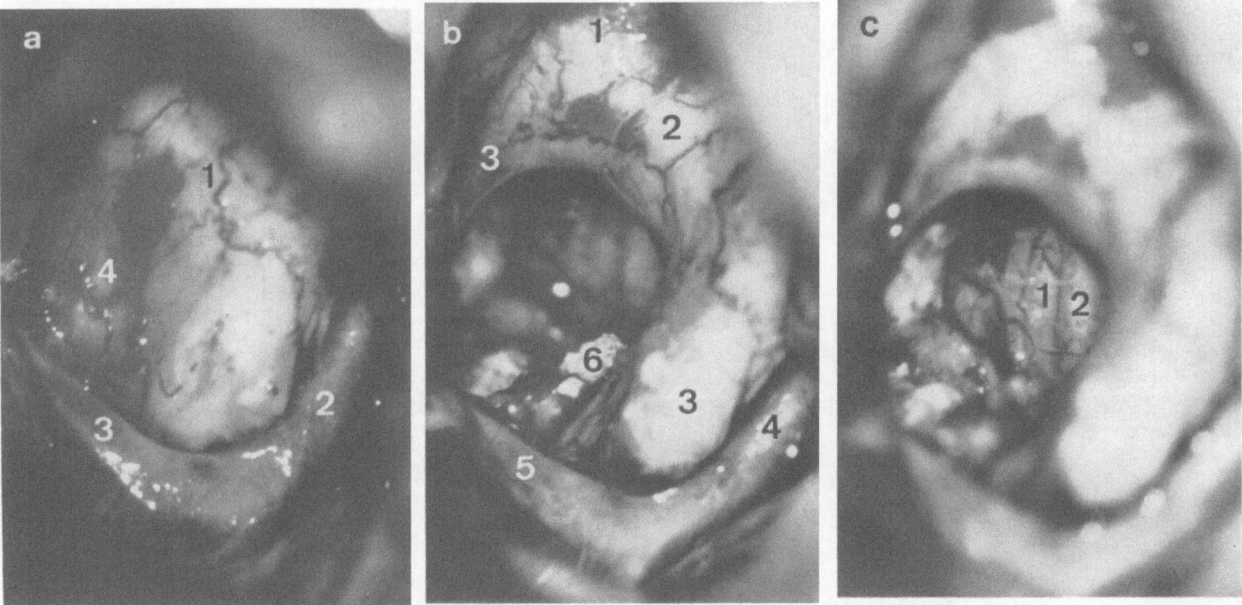

Fig. 6a–c. Suprasellar retrochiasmal partially cystic craniopharyngioma (prefixed chiasm). a) Through a subfrontal approach, the prefixed optic chiasm (*1*), the right internal carotid artery (*2*), the anterior cerebral artery (*3*) and the lamina terminalis (*4*) are exposed. b) Operative view after the lamina terminalis has been opened. The short left optic nerve (*1*), the chiasm (*2*), both optic tracts (*3*), the right internal carotid artery (*4*) and the anterior cerebral artery (*5*) are visualized. A small portion of tumor tissue in the anterior inferior portion of the third ventricle and the retrosellar region are visualized (*6*). c) View after total tumor removal. The microscope is focused on the deeper structured in the retrosellar region, the oculomotor nerve (*1*) and the posterior communicating artery (*2*) are visualized

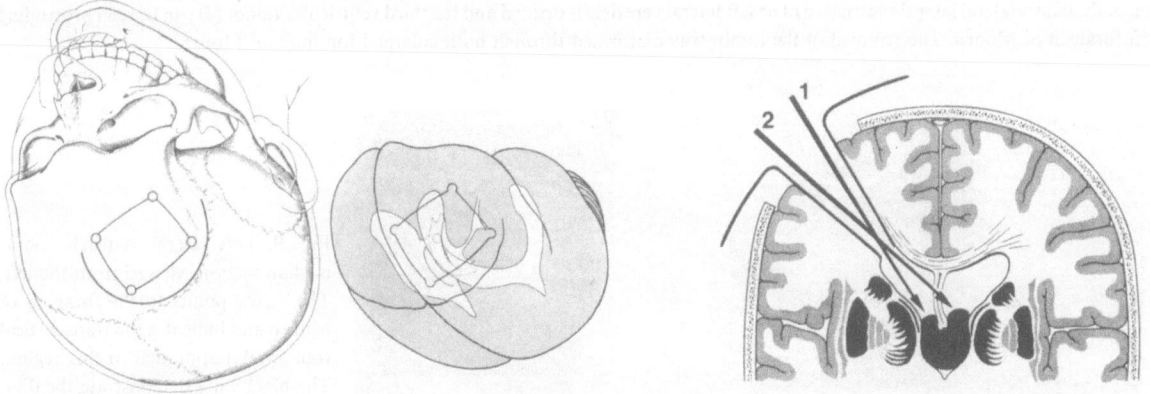

Fig. 7. Schematic presentation of the transcortical transfrontal approach (left) and the transfrontal transventricular approaches (right) (see Table 1). *1* Transfrontal transventricular transforaminal approach, *2* transfrontal transventricular transseptal approach

result in a disconnection syndrome with impairment of visual motor coordination. Therefore, this route should only be used for infiltrating tumors located in the pulvinar region of the thalamus which are associated with a significant neurological deficit or limited life expectancy.

Problems Related to the Division of the Fornix and the Anterior Commissure[5, 8, 19, 20, 25, 27, 73, 80, 91, 96, 98]

As after section of the anterior corpus callosum, we did not see any post-operative deficits attributable to compromise of the anterior column of a single fornix by anterior enlargement of the foramen of Monro. It

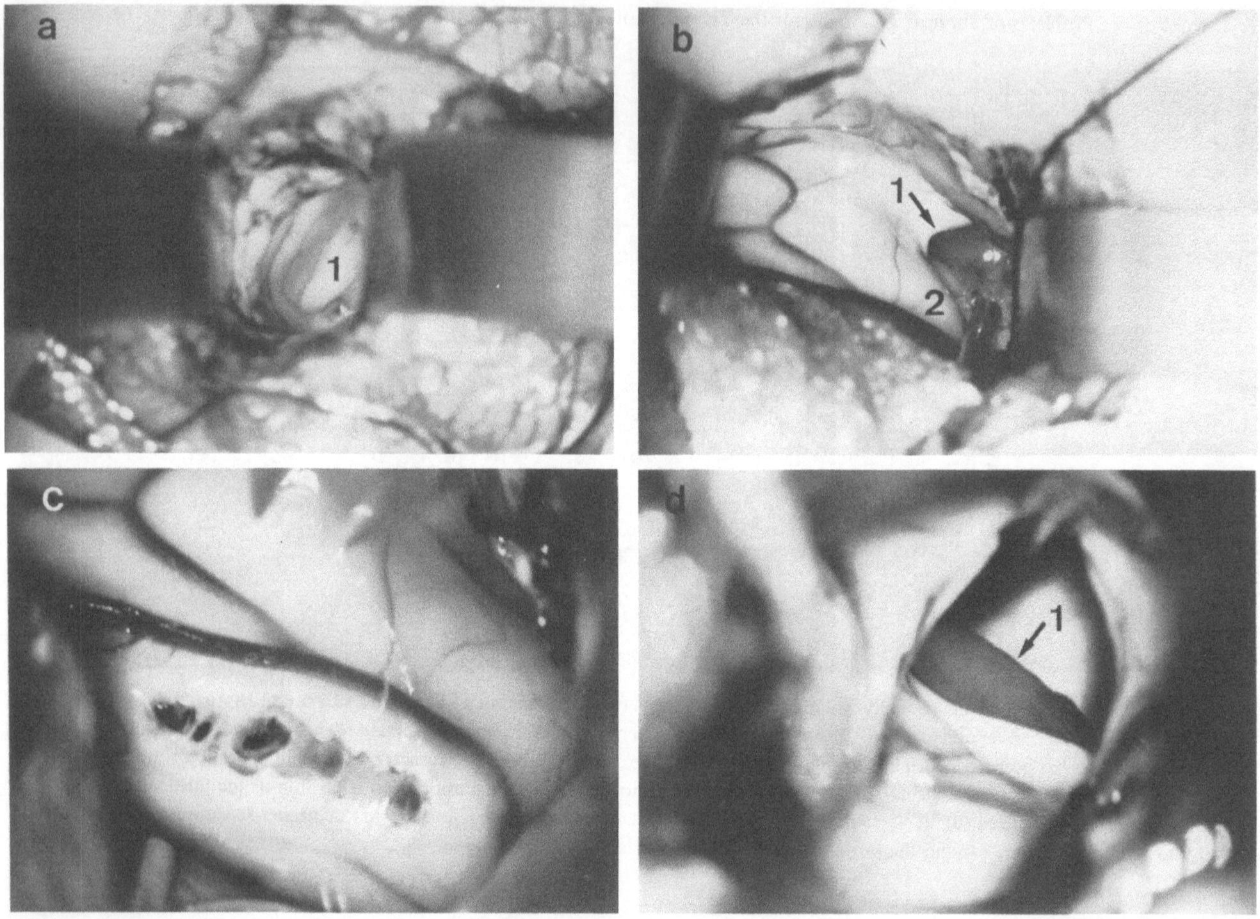

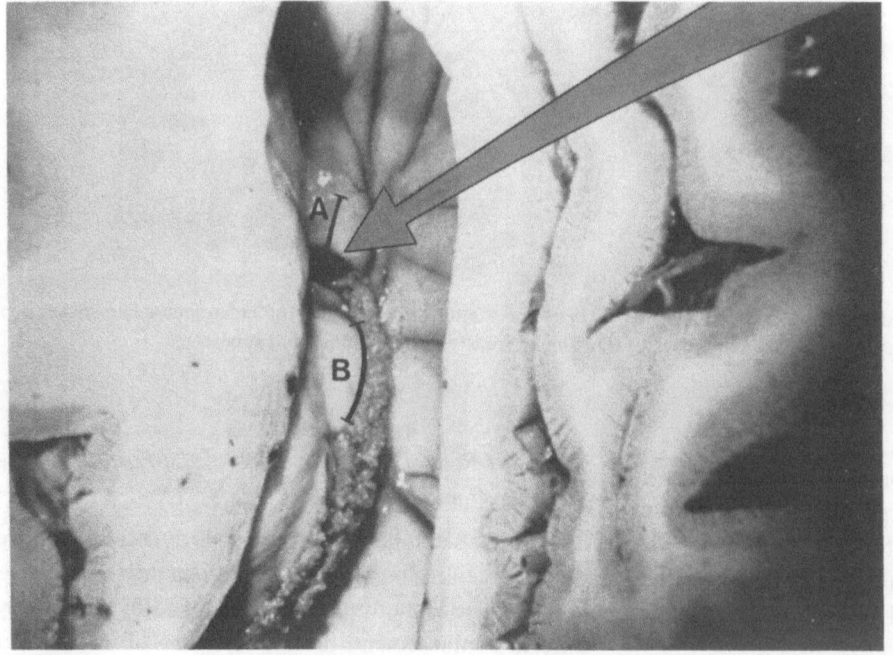

Fig. 8a–d. Ependymoma within the anterior part of the third ventricle. The tumor protrudes slightly through both foramina of Monro into the lateral ventricles. a) Through a transcortical transfrontal approach the right lateral ventricle is entered and the bulging septum pellucidum (*1*) is visualized. b) The foramen of Monro (*1*) has been exposed. The septal vein and the choroid plexus (*2*) were used as a guide to locate the foramen of Monro which was not immediately visible. The tumor is seen through the foramen. c) Incision of the distended septum pellucidum allows visualization of the contralateral lateral ventricle. d) The left lateral ventricle is opened and the third ventricular tumor (*1*) can be seen protruding from the left foramen of Monro. The removal of the tumor was performed through both enlarged foramina of Monro

Fig. 9. Left lateral ventricle, paramedian section, viewed from the left. The arrow points to the foramen of Monro and indicates the transcortical transfrontal approach to this region. The black lines demonstrate the division of the anterior column of the fornix (*A*), and the opening of the lateral portion of the roof of the third ventricle (*B*). The latter "subchoroidal" approach can be accomplished after the choroid plexus has been elevated and retracted medially, and small leptomeningeal vessels of the tela choroidea have been coagulated; then the tela choroidea can be divided. The thalamostriate vein may be divided, but with precaution not to damage the internal cerebral vein

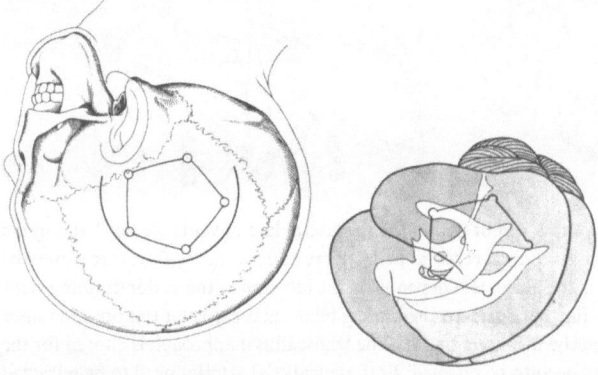

Fig. 10. Schematic presentation of the transcortical transparietal transventricular approach (see Table 1)

should be stressed that in all these patients the transcortical transventricular approach was chosen. Particular care was taken not to lacerate the contralateral fornix and the anterior commissure. Basically, the authors avoid the method of dividing the anterior column of the fornix to gain easy access to the contents of the anterior third ventricle.

Problems Related to Division of the Thalamostriate Vein[8, 30, 73]

Although division of the thalamostriate vein is practiced by several surgeons, its safety has not yet been established. Depending on the anatomical variation of this vein its interruption may be without consequences, but may also cause severe motor and sensory deficits secondary to hemorrhagic infarction of the basal ganglia.

Problems Related to Compression of the Anterior Part of the Sagittal Sinus[8, 42, 84, 88]

Problems have been encountered on forceful retraction of the superior sagittal sinus which has resulted in deficits of frontal lobe function, and when injuring both fornices or the septal region which has resulted in akinetic mutism.

Surgical Mortality

In our experience with patients encompassing all types of third ventricular tumors, surgical mortality was below 5%. Approximately 30% of the tumors were benign, encapsulated, and resectable.

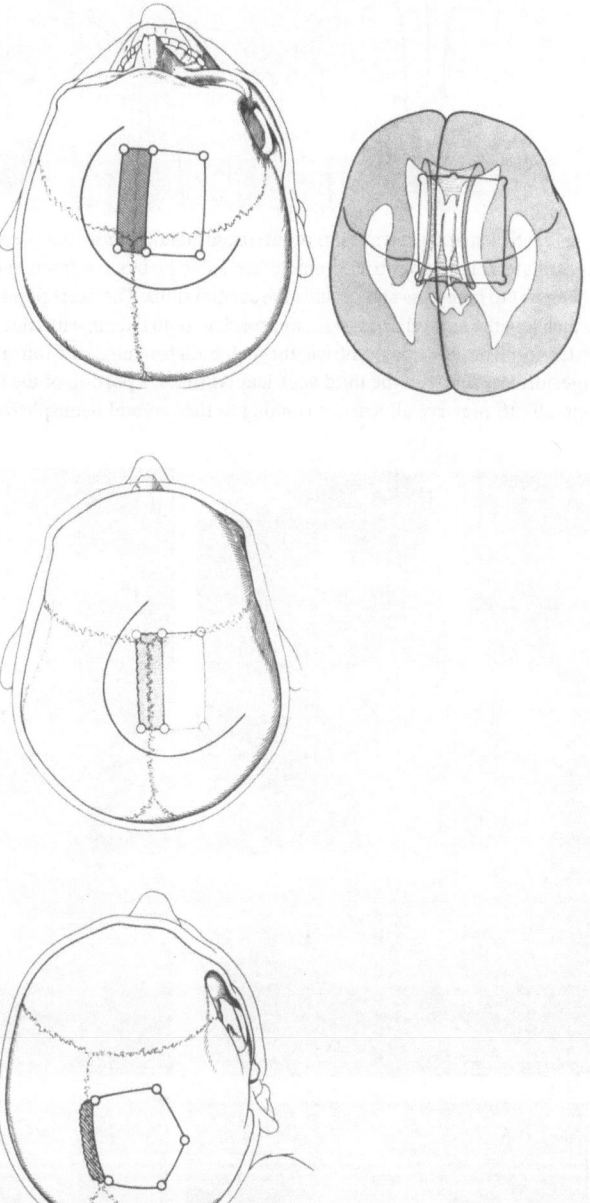

Fig. 11. Schematic presentation of the various midline interhemispheric transcallosal approaches (see Table 1): Anterior transcallosal approach (above), middle transcallosal approach (middle), and posterior transcallosal approach (below)

Conclusion

Because of the uncertainty of a histological diagnosis without biopsy in tumors which lie within the third ventricle, we have advocated surgical exploration of all cases. Given advanced techniques of neuroradiology, neuroanesthesiology, microneurosurgery, sophisticated pre- and post-operative intensive care, and recently improved understanding of micro-

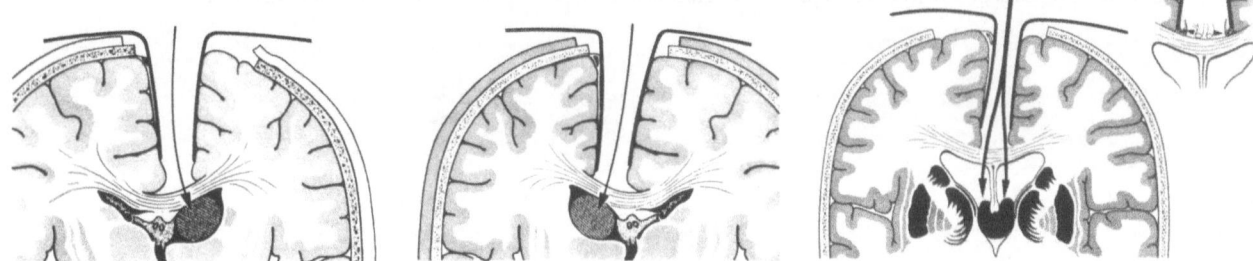

Fig. 12. Schematic presentation of interhemispheric transcallosal approaches to a tumor within the ipsilateral lateral ventricle (left) and in the contralateral lateral ventricle (middle, see Table 1). Upon retraction of the contralateral cerebral hemisphere along with the falx, care should be taken not to compress and occlude the sagittal sinus. The exact point of retractor placement depends on the location of the major draining veins which join the sagittal sinus.—An approach to both lateral ventricles (right) may be considered in cases of bilateral ventricular tumors and tumor extension from the third ventricle through both foramina of Monro. An interhemispheric but midline transcallosal approach is chosen for the interfornical access to the third ventricle. At times, a portion of the falx may need to be resected. Both pericallosal arteries need to be retracted laterally to preserve all arteries running to the cerebral hemispheres

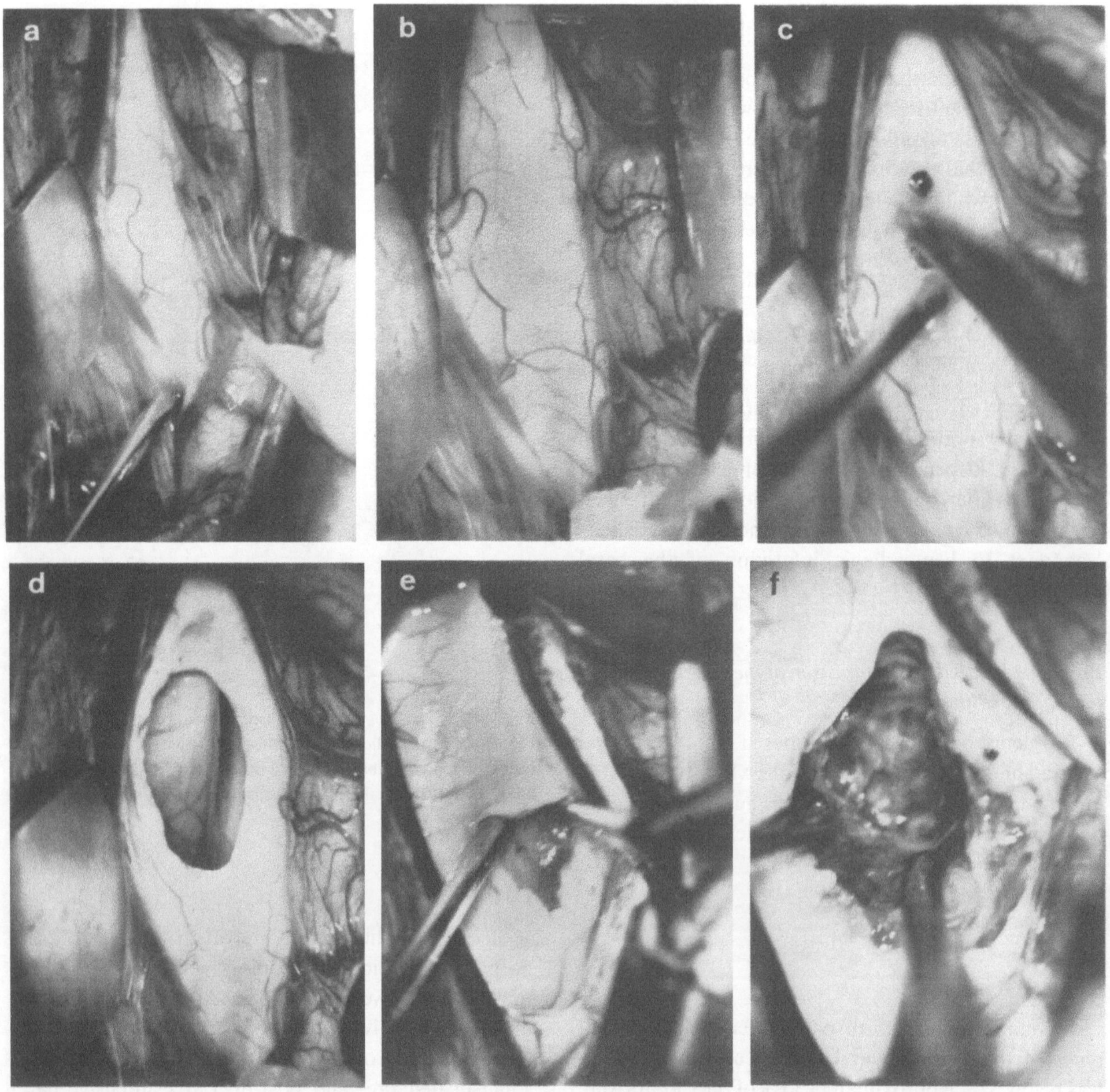

Fig. 13 a–f. Astrocytoma of the third ventricle. Midline interhemispheric transcallosal approach. a) The right cerebral hemisphere has been retracted laterally, the falx has been moderately retracted medially. b) The white corpus callosum is exposed. c) The midline of the corpus callosum has been incised. d) The right lateral ventricle is seen through the opening in the corpus callosum. The body of the fornix is stretched over the third ventricle. e) The third ventricle is opened between the bodies of the stretched out fornices. f) astrocytoma is exposed within the third ventricle

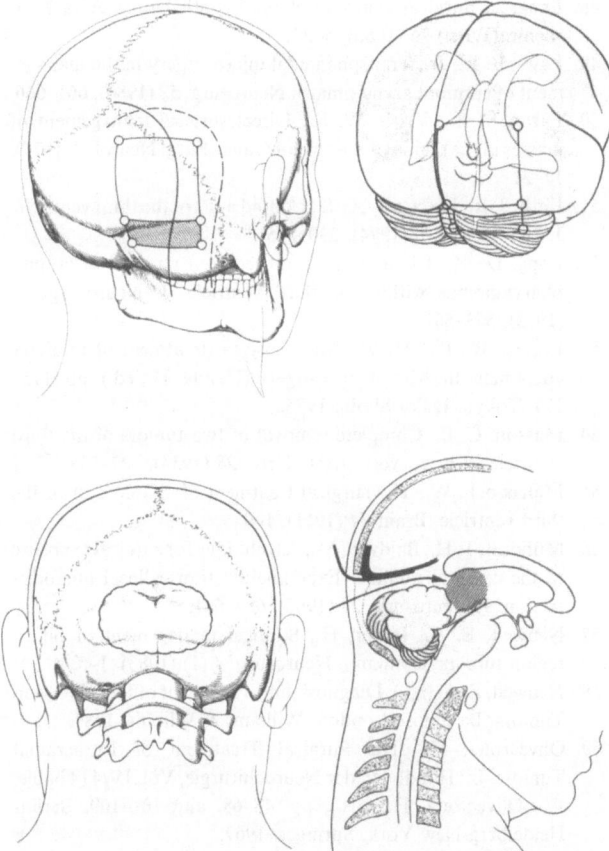

Fig. 14. Schematic presentation of the commonly used "posterior" approaches to midline lesions in the pineal and quadrigeminal plate region (see Table 1). Occipital transtentorial approach (above) and infratentorial supracerebellar approach (below). The illustrated approaches are performed with the patient in the sitting position. For the infratentorial supracerebellar approach the bony removal must extend up to the confluens sinuum (torcular) and above the transverse sinus. The latter anatomical structures can gently be elevated by retractor to allow an excellent view during the further approach to the pineal region and the posterior third ventricle

neuroanatomy and -topography of the CNS, etc., the authors would think there is very little justification for delaying a direct approach of such lesions.

References

1. Antunes, J. K., Muraszko, K., Quest, D. O., Carmel, P. W., Surgical strategies in the management of tumours of the anterior third ventricle. In: Modern Neurosurgery 1 (Brock, E. M., ed.), pp. 215–224. Berlin-Heidelberg-New York: Springer. 1982.
2. Apuzzo, M. L. V., Transcallosal interfornical exposure of lesions of the third ventricle. In: Operative Neurosurgical Techniques, Vol. 1 (Schmidek, H. H., Sweet, W. H., eds.), pp. 585–594, New York-London: Grune and Stratton. 1982.
3. Apuzzo, M. L. V., Chikovani, O., Gott, P., Transcallosal, interfornical approaches for lesions affecting the third ventricle: Surgical considerations and consequences. Neurosurgery *10* (1982), 547–554.
4. Baldwin, M., Ommaya, A. K., Farrier, R., Mesial cerebral incision. J. Neurosurg. *20* (1963), 679–686.
5. Bengochea, F. G., De la Torre, O., Esquivel, O., The section of the fornix in the surgical treatment of certain epilepsies. Trans. Am. Neurol. Assoc. *79* (1959), 176–178.
6. Brunner, C., cited in: Rorschach, H., Zur Pathologie der Tumoren der Zirbeldrüse. Beitr. Klin. Chir. *83* (1913), 451.
7. Busch, E., A new approach for the removal of tumors of the third ventricle. Acta Psychiat. *19* (1944), 57–60.
8. Carmel, P. W., Tumors of the third ventricle. Acta Neurochir. (Wien) *75* (1985), 136–146.
9. Clark, K., The occipital transtentorial approach to the pineal region. In: Operative Neurosurgical Techniques, Vol. 1 (Schmidek, H. H., Sweet, W. H., eds.), pp. 595–597. New York-London: Grune & Stratton. 1982.
10. Dandy, W. E., An operation for the removal of pineal tumors. Surg. Gynec. Obstet. *33* (1921), 113–119.
11. Dandy, W. E., Diagnosis, localization and removal of tumors of the third ventricle. Johns Hopkins Hospital Bulletin *33* (1923), 188–194.
12. Dandy, W. E., Benign Tumors in the Third Ventricle of the Brain. Diagnosis and Treatment. Springfield, Ill.: Ch. C Thomas. 1933.
13. Dandy, W. E., Surgery of the Brain. In: Lewis' Practice of Surgery, Vol. 12. Hagerstown, Maryland: Prior Co. 1945.
14. Dandy, W. E., Operative experience in cases of pineal tumor. Arch. Surg. *33* (1936), 16–46.
15. Diamond, S. J., Scammell, R. E., Brouwers, E. Y. M., Weeks, R., Functions of the centre section (trunk) of the corpus callosum in man. Brain *100* (1977), 543–562.
16. Foerster, O., Ein Fall von Vierhügeltumor, durch Operation entfernt. Arch. Psychiat. Nervenkr. *84* (1928), 515–516.
17. Foerster, O., Das operative Vorgehen bei Tumoren der Vierhügelgegend. Wien. Klin. Wschr. *41* (1928), 986–990.
18. Foerster, O., Über das operative Vorgehen bei Operationen der Vierhügelgegend. Zbl. Ges. Neurol. Psychiat. *61* (1932), 457–459.
19. Fujii, K., Lenkey, C., Rhoton, A. L., r., Microsurgical anatomy of the choroidal arteries: Lateral and third ventricles. J. Neurosurg. *52* (1980), 165–188.
20. Gazzaniga, M. S., Risse, G. L., Springer, S. P., Clark, E., Wilson, D. H., Psychologic and neurologic consequences of partial and complete cerebral commissurotomy. Neurology *25* (1975), 10–15.
21. Geffen, G., Walsh, A., Simpson, D., Jeeves, M., Comparison of the effects of transcortical and transcallosal removal of intraventricular tumors. Brain *103* (1980), 773–788.
22. Glasauer, F. E., An operative approach to pineal tumors. Acta Neurochir. (Wien) *22* (1970), 177–180.
23. Halstead, A. E., Remarks on the operative treatment of tumors of the hypophysis. Surg. Gynec. Obstet. *10* (1910), 494–502.
24. Hamberger, C. A., Hammer, G., Norlen, G., Sjörgren, B., Surgical treatment of craniopharyngioma: Radical removal by the transantro-sphenoidal approach. Acta Otolaryngol. (Stockholm) *52* (1960), 285–292.
25. Hardy, J., Vezina, J. L., Transphenoidal neurosurgery of intracranial neoplasm. Adv. Neurol. *15* (1976), 261–274.

26. Hassler, R., Riechert, T., Über einen Fall von doppelseitiger Fornicotomie bei sogenannter temporaler Epilepsie. Acta Neurochir. (Wien) 5 (1957), 330–340.

27. Heilmann, K. M., Sypert, G. W., Korsakoff's syndrome resulting from bilateral fornix lesions. Neurology 27 (1977), 490-493.

28. Heppner, F., Zur Operationstechnik bei Pinealomen. Zbl. Neurochir. 19 (1959), 219–224.

29. Heppner, F., Operative Zugangswege bei Pinealomen. In: Pädiatrische Neurochirurgie (Kraus, H., Sunder-Plassmann, M., eds.), pp. 273–275. Wien: Verlag der Wiener Med. Akademie. 1970.

30. Hirsch, J. F., Zouaoui, A., Renier, D., Pierre-Kahn, A., A new surgical approach to the third ventricle with interruption of the striothalamic vein. Acta Neurochir. (Wien) 47 (1979), 135–147.

31. Hoff, H., Schönbauer, L., Hirnchirurgie: Erfahrungen und Resultate, pp. 398–402. Leipzig-Wien: F. Deuticke. 1933.

32. Horrax., G., Extirpation of a large pinealoma from a patient with pubertas precox: a new operative approach. Arch. Neurol. Psychiat. 37 (1937), 385–397.

33. Jamieson, K. G., Excision of pineal tumors. J. Neurosurg. 35 (1971), 550–553.

34. Jeeves, M. A., Simpson, D. A., Geffen, G., Functional consequences of the transcallosal removal of intraventricular tumors. J. Neurol. Neurosurg. Psychiat. 42 (1979), 134–142.

35. Kempe, L. G., Operative Neurosurgery. Vol. I: Cranial, Cerebral and Intracranial Vascular Diseases, pp. 1–21, and 145–155. Berlin-Heidelberg-New York: Springer. 1968.

36. King, T. T., Removal of intraventricular craniopharyngiomas through the lamina terminalis. Acta Neurochir. (Wien) 45 (1979), 277–286.

37. Konovalov, A. N., Operative management of craniopharyngiomas. In: Advances and Technical Standards in Neurosurgery, Vol. 8 (Krayenbühl, H., *et al.*, eds.), pp. 281–318. Wien-New York: Springer. 1981.

38. Konovalov, A. N., Microsurgery of craniopharyngiomas. In: Microneurosurgery (Rand, R. W., ed.), pp. 196–213. St. Louis-Toronto-Princetown: C. V. Mosby. 1985.

39. Koos, W. T., Miller, M. H., Intracranial Tumors of Infants and Children. Stuttgart: Thieme. 1971.

40. Koos, W. T., Böck, F. W., Salah, S., Experiences in the microsurgery of craniopharyngiomas. In: Microneurosurgery (Handa, H., ed.), pp. 151–160. Tokyo: Igaku Shoin. 1975.

41. Koos, W. T., Böck, F. W., Spetzler, R. F., (eds.), Clinical Microneurosurgery. Stuttgart: Thieme. 1976.

42. Koos, W. T., Spetzler, R. F., Pendl, G., Perneczky, A., Lang, J., Color Atlas of Microneurosurgery. Stuttgart-New York: Thieme; New York: Thieme & Stratton. 1985.

43. Krause, F., Chirurgie des Gehirns und Rückenmarks. Vol. 1, pp. 82–84, and Vol. 2, pp. 548–552. Berlin-Wien: Urban & Schwarzenberg. 1908 (Vol. 1), 1911 (Vol. 2).

44. Krause, F., Freilegung des Pons, Oberwurm und der Vierhügel. In: Die allgemeine Chirurgie der Gehirnkrankheiten (Krause, F., ed.). Stuttgart: Enke. 1914.

45. Krause, F., Operative Freilegung der Vierhügel, nebst Beobachtungen über Hirndruck und Dekompression. Zbl. Chirurgie 53 (1926), 2812–2819.

46. Kunicki, A., Operative experiences in 8 cases of pineal tumor. J. Neurosurg. 17 (1960), 815–823.

47. Lang, J., Clinical Anatomy of the Head. Neurocranium—Orbit—Craniocervical Regions. Berlin-Heidelberg-New York: Springer. 1983.

48. Lang, J., Surgical anatomy of the hypothalamus. Acta Neurochir. (Wien) 75 (1985), 5–22.

49. Laws, E. R., Jr., Transphenoidal microsurgery in the management of craniopharyngioma. J. Neurosurg. 52 (1980), 661–666.

50. Lazar, M. L., Vlark, W. K., Direct surgical management of masses in the region of the vein of Galen. Surg. Neurol. 2 (1974), 17–21.

51. Little, J. R., MacCarty, C. S., Colloid cysts of the third ventricle. J. Neurosurg. 40 (1974), 230–235.

52. Long, D. M., Chou, S. N., Transcallosal removal of craniopharyngiomas within the third ventricle. J. Neurosurg. 39 (1973), 563–567.

53. Lorenz, R., Pia, H. W., Microsurgical treatment of pituitary adenomas. In: Microneurosurgery (Handa, H., ed.), pp. 173–177. Tokyo: Igaku Shoin. 1975.

54. Masson, C. B., Complete removal of two tumors of the third ventricle with recovery. Arch. Surg. 28 (1934), 527–537.

55. McKissock, W., The surgical treatment of colloid cyst of the third ventricle. Brain 74 (1951), 1–9.

56. Milhorat, T. H., Baldwin, M., A technique for surgical exposure of the cerebral midline: Experimental transcallosal microdissection. J. Neurosurg. 24 (1966), 687–691.

57. Neuwelt, E. A., Batjer, H., Surgical management of pineal region tumors. Contemp. Neurosurg. 4 (1) (1983), 1–5.

58. Neuwelt, E. A. (ed.), Diagnosis and Treatment of Pineal Region Tumors. Baltimore-London: Williams & Wilkins. 1984.

59. Olivecrona, H., The Surgical Treatment of Intracranial Tumors. In: Handbuch der Neurochirurgie, Vol. IV/4 (Tönnis, W., Olivecrona, H., eds.), pp. 48–68, and 101–109. Berlin-Heidelberg-New York: Springer. 1967.

60. Oppenheim, H., Krause, F., Operative Erfolge bei Geschwülsten der Sehhügel- und Vierhügelgegend. Berlin. Klin. Wschr. 50 (1913), 2316–2322.

61. Page, L. K., The infratentorial-supracerebellar exposure of tumors in the pineal area. Neurosurgery 1 (1977), 36–40.

62. Pendl, G., Infratentorial approach to mesencephalic tumors. In: Clinical Microneurosurgery (Koos, W. T., Böck, F. W., Spetzler, R. F., eds.), pp. 143–150. Stuttgart: Thieme. 1976.

63. Pendl, G., Koos, W. T., Witzmann, A., Surgical approach to pineal tumors in childhood. Z. Kinderchir. 34 (1981), 203–204.

64. Pendl, G., The surgery of pineal lesions. In: Diagnosis and Treatment of Pineal Region Tumors (Neuwelt, E. A., ed.), pp. 139–154. Baltimore-London: Williams & Wilkins. 1984.

65. Pendl, G., Microsurgical Anatomy of the Pineal Region. In: Diagnosis and Treatment of Pineal Region Tumors (Neuwelt, E. A., ed.), pp. 155–207. Baltimore-London: Williams & Wilkins. 1984.

66. Poppen, J. L., An Atlas of Neurosurgical Technique. Philadelphia: W. B. Saunders. 1960.

67. Poppen, J. L., The right occipital approach to a pinealoma. J. Neurosurg. 25 (1966), 706–710.

68. Poppen, J. L., Marino, R., Jr., Pinealomas and tumors of the posterior portion of the third ventricle. J. Neurosurg. 28 (1968), 357–364.

69. Poppen, J. L., Reyes, V., Horrax, G., Colloid cysts of the third ventricle. J. Neurosurg. 10 (1953), 242–263.

70. Rand, R. W., Transfrontal transphenoidal craniotomy in pituitary and related tumors. In: Microneurosurgery (Rand, R. W., ed.), pp. 93–104. St. Louis: Mosby. 1978.

71. Reid, W. S., Clark, W. K., Comparison of the intratentorial and transtentorial approaches to the pineal region. Neurosurgery 3 (1978), 1–8.

72. Rhoton, A. L., Jr., Hardy, D. G., Chambers, S. M., Microsurgical anatomy and dissection of the sphenoid bone, cavernous sinus and sellar region. Surg. Neurol. *12* (1979), 63–104.

73. Rhoton, A. L. Jr., Yamamoto, I., Peace, D. A., Microsurgery of the third ventricle. Part 2: Operative approaches. Neurosurgery *8* (1981), 357–373.

74. Rorschach, H., Zur Pathologie der Tumoren und der Operabilität der Zirbeldrüse. Beitr. Klin. Chir. *83* (1913), 451.

75. Sano, K., Diagnosis and treatment of tumors in the pineal region. Acta Neurochir. (Wien) *34* (1976), 153–157.

76. Sano, K., Microsurgery of tumors in the pineal region. In: Microneurosurgery (Rand, R. W., ed.), pp. 391–397. St. Louis-Toronto-Princetown: C. V. Mosby. 1985.

77. Scarff, J. E., Third ventriculostomy by puncture of the lamina terminalis and the floor of the third ventricle. J. Neurosurg. *24* (1966), 935–943.

78. Schmidek, H. H., Brady, I. W., De Vita, V. T., (eds.), Pineal Tumors. New York: Masson Publishing U.S.A. Inc. 1977.

79. Schürmann, K., Die Neurochirurgie der intrakraniellen Tumoren der Mittellinie. Radiologie *5* (1965), 459–473.

80. Seeger, W., Microsurgery of the Brain: Anatomical and Technical Principles, Vol. 1, pp. 56–171, and pp. 286–341. Wien-New York: Springer. 1980.

81. Shucart, W. A., Stein, B. M., Transcallosal approach to the anterior ventricular system. Neurosurgery *3* (1978), 339–343.

82. Spencer, D. D., Collins, W. F., Surgical management of lateral intraventricular tumors. In: Operative Neurosurgical Techniques, Vol. 1 (Schmidek, H. H., Sweet, W. H., eds.), pp. 561–574. New York-London: Grune & Stratton. 1982.

83. Stein, B. M., The infratentorial supracerebellar approach to pineal lesions. J. Neurosurg. *35* (1971), 197–202.

84. Stein, B. M., Transcallosal approach to third ventricle tumors. In: Current Techniques in Operative Neurosurgery (Schmidek, H. H., Sweet, W. H., eds.), pp. 247–255. New York: Grune & Stratton. 1977.

85. Stein, B. M., Supracerebellar approach for pineal region neoplasms. In: Current Techniques in Operative Neurosurgery (Schmidek, H. H., Sweet, W. H., eds.), pp. 257–264. New York: Grune & Stratton. 1977.

86. Stein, B. M., Supracerebellar-infratentorial approach to pineal tumors. Surg. Neurol. *11* (1979), 331–337.

87. Stein, B. M., Surgical treatment of pineal tumors. Clin. Neurosurg. *26* (1979), 490–510.

88. Stein, B. M., Transcallosal approach to third ventricular tumors. In: Operative Neurosurgical Techniques, Vol. 1 (Schmidek, H. H., Sweet, W. H., eds.), pp. 575–584. New York-London: Grune & Stratton. 1982.

89. Stein, B. M., Supracerebellar approach for pineal region neoplasms. In: Operative Neurosurgical Techniques, Vol. 1 (Schmidek, H. H., Sweet, W. H., eds.), pp. 599–607. New York-London: Grune & Stratton. 1982.

90. Sweet, W. H., Craniopharyngiomas, with a note on Rathke's cleft or epithelial cysts and on suprasellar cysts. In: Operative Neurosurgical Techniques, Vol. 1 (Schmidek, H. H., Sweet, W. H., eds.), pp. 291–325. New York-London: Grune & Stratton. 1982.

91. Sweet, W. H., Talland, G. A., Ervin, F. R., Loss of recent memory following section of fornix. Trans. Am. Neurol. Assoc. *84* (1959), 76–82.

92. Symon, L., The intracranial approach to tumors in the area of the sella turcica. In: Operative Surgery: Neurosurgery (Symon, L., ed.), pp. 181–186. London: Butterworth. 1979.

93. Van Wagenen, W. P., A surgical approach for the removal of certain pineal tumors. Surg. Gynec. Obstet. *53* (1931), 216–220.

94. Viale, G. L., Turtas, S., The subchoroid approach to the third ventricle. Surg. Neurol. *14* (1980), 71–76.

95. Winston, K. R., Cavazzuti, V., Arkins, T., Absence of neurological and behavioral abnormalities after anterior transcallosal operation for third ventricle lesions. Neurosurgery *4* (1979), 386–393.

96. Woolsey, R. O., Nelson, J. S., Asymptomatic destruction of the fornix in man. Arch. Neurol. *32* (1975), 566–568.

97. Yamamoto, I., Rhoton, A. L., Peace, D. A., Microsurgery of the third ventricle, Part 1: Microsurgical anatomy. Neurosurgery *8* (1981), 334–356.

98. Zaidel, D., Sperry, R. W., Memory impairment after commissurotomy in man. Brain *97* (1974), 263–272.

99. Zapletal, B., Ein operativer Zugang zum Gebiet der Incisura tentorii. Zbl. Neurochir. *16* (1956), 64–69.

100. Zülch, K. J., Brain Tumors. New York: Springer. 1957.

Authors' address: W. Th. Koos, M.D., Professor of Neurosurgery, Department of Neurosurgery, University of Vienna Medical School, Währinger Gürtel 18-20, A-1090 Wien, Austria.

Acta Neurochirurgica, Suppl. 35, 42–49 (1985)
© by Springer-Verlag 1985

Operative Approaches to Midline Tumors

B. M. Stein

Department of Neurological Surgery, College of Physicians and Surgeons of Columbia University, New York, N.Y, U.S.A.

Summary

We have now operated and confirmed 80 tumors of the pineal region. Our experience is that 30 percent of these are benign, encapsulated and can be removed, and that only 30 percent represent germinomas. Another 30 percent are astrocytomas of varying grade. The preferred therapy in the majority of these tumors is radiotherapy and its extent depends upon the analysis of the lumbar spinal fluid. Chemotherapy has been reserved for tumors of the primitive embryonic type.

The result of surgery for benign tumors has been excellent and the recurrence rate extremely low. In the germinoma series, the response to radiation therapy in our experience has been promising initially with resolution of the tumor by CT scan. However, we have noted recurrence of some of these tumors after radiotherapy approximately 6 to 8 years after the institution of therapy. The pineoblastomas are extremely difficult to treat by whatever means and the same holds true for the malignant pineocytomas. Our experience is too limited to say what the outcome will be in the chemotherapeutic management of the more primitive and embryonal tumors.

Keywords: Midline brain tumors; third ventricle; pineal region; approaches.

Introduction

In this discussion I will confine my remarks to midline approaches to third ventricular tumors and will not discuss other pathology occurring within the third ventricle. Emphasis will be placed primarily on those tumors approached through the dorsal anterior third ventricle and through the pineal route. Although anatomically the borders of the third ventricle encompass a small region of the brain, the obscure location of the third ventricle requires three different surgical approaches in order to cope with the tumors that occupy this region.

A wide range of tumor types requires[3,14] (1) histological identification prior to treatment, and (2) therapy tailored to the nature of the lesions. The use of the operation microscope and microsurgical techniques has permitted exposure of these tumors, resection of benign (encapsulated) tumors and identification with possible debulking of invasive (infiltrative) tumors with a high degree of safety. Small exposures with minimal brain retraction are possible through the use of the operation microscope. Furthermore, these profound regions of the brain are visualized with excellent illumination not heretofore obtained. The surgical approaches are designed for the microscope and microsurgical techniques and should not be performed without these.

Basic Surgical Approaches

The borders of the third ventricle as observed in the sagittal plane from the right side can be correlated to the face of a clock. Furthermore, the third ventricle should be regionalized to the following: 1) anterior middorsal or foramen of Monro region—12 to 4 o'clock, 2) anteroposterior or chiasmatic—4 to 8 o'clock, and 3) posterior third ventricle—8 to 12 o'clock.

(A) Anteroposterior

The standard subfrontal exposures with minor modification are used to expose tumors located in this region of the third ventricle. Through the use of the operation microscope and microsurgical instrumentation with self-retaining retractors bifrontal exposures are no longer necessary. This area may be exposed via the pterional approach almost always from the non-

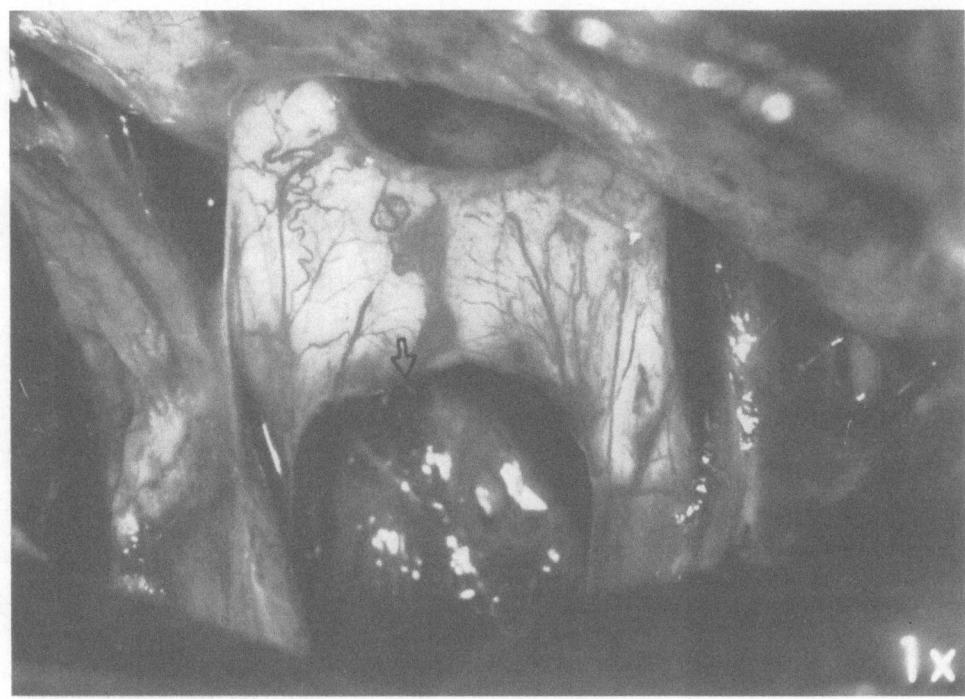

Fig. 1. Operative photograph of right subfrontal exposure showing a craniopharyngioma (arrow) visualized through a wide open lamina terminalis. The arrow overlies the left side of the chiasm

dominant hemisphere. Upon opening the arachnoid of the chiasm, gliomas of the chiasm or hypothalamus may be visualized and resected or biopsied. To enter the third ventricle, more extensive retraction must be used to expose the lamina terminalis—the route to this area of the third ventricle (Fig.1). The anterior cerebral and anterior communicating arteries will be subjected to the most retraction and manipulation via this route. Care must be taken not to injure or occlude these arteries. The lamina terminalis may be opened fully; even so, angulation and the limitation of the opening permit only a limited view of the third ventricle. Necessary dissection around benign tumors that are adherent to the ventricular wall may be impossible and only partial removal of the tumor may be accomplished via this route. Because of this I have not extensively used the route.

(B) Anterior–Middorsal Region

The prime route of entry into this portion of the third ventricle is through the foramen of Monro. This is best approached through one of two routes: (1) trans-cortical (frontal) incision directly to the lateral ventricle or (2) transcallosal incision to either or both lateral

ventricles. Since I prefer the latter route, it will be discussed in some detail[15,16]. The target of this route is the anterior one-third of the corpus callosum. The patient is positioned in the sitting/slouch position, well padded and supported. As with any operation in the sitting position, Doppler monitoring is essential in order to detect air embolism early. The patient's head is held rigidly in a pin vise headholder in a position which results in the skull at the coronal suture being horizontal. The scalp flap will be "U" shaped or curvilinear on the right side. A triangular bone flap based over the midline slightly to the left is formed and need not be large. One-third of the bone flap is behind the coronal suture and two-thirds in front. The dura is reflected toward the midline and all bridging veins anterior to the coronal suture are cauterized and sacrificed to permit lateral retraction of the frontal lobe.

The brain should be decompressed by shunting or ventricular drainage and the frontal lobe retracted away from the falx gradually. The first pitfall is now encountered- the cingulate gyrus as it is adherent to its opposite beneath the falx may be mistaken by the inexperienced surgeon for the corpus callosum. Its cortical appearance as opposed to the stark white nature of the corpus callosum should settle the issue.

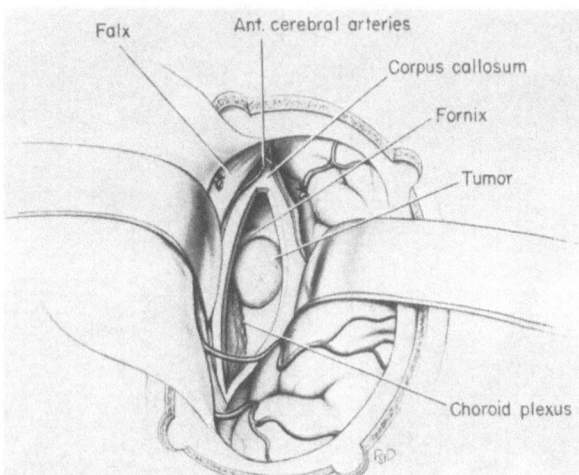

Fig. 2. Drawing of the transcallosal exposure used for access to the lateral and third ventricles. The drawing shows all of the essential landmarks of this operative procedure with the tumor protruding from the region of the right foramen of Monro

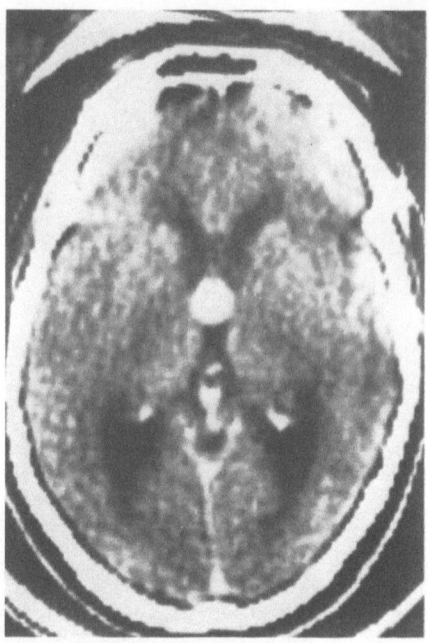

Fig. 3A. CT scan showing dense contrast enhancement of a colloid cyst of the third ventricle

The cistern over the corpus callosum is opened and the anterior cerebral arteries separated using microsurgical techniques with the operation microscope. Rarely are the anterior cerebral arteries so convoluted and inter-twined that it is necessary to go to one or the other side of both of these arteries. Usually the exposure is between the two major trunks. An elliptical area about 2.5 cms long of the corpus callosum is removed by suction cautery until the ependyma is encountered. When all of the ependymal lining of this area of resection has been exposed, the ependymal veins may be cauterized and the ependyma opened directly. At this point, there is possible entry into three structures either lateral ventricle or a cavum septum pellucidum. In the latter instance, the situation is confusing until the surgeon realizes that he cannot visualize any of the structures associated with a normal lateral ventricle. When entry has been made into a lateral ventricle, the following structure should be identified for anatomical reference (Fig. 2): 1) choroid plexus, 2) thalamostriate vein, and 3) septal vein. When these are located it is then possible to identify the foramen of Monro and the interventricular septum. Tumors of the third ventricle usually cause the foramen of Monro to dilate.

The major issue to be addressed at this point deals with the opening of the foramen of Monro in order to provide room for removal of third ventricular tumors. This may be done in three ways: 1) cutting one fornix anteriorly, 2) subchoroidal opening along the dorsal part of the thalamus with division of the thalamostriate vein, 3) retraction and preservation of the fornix. When

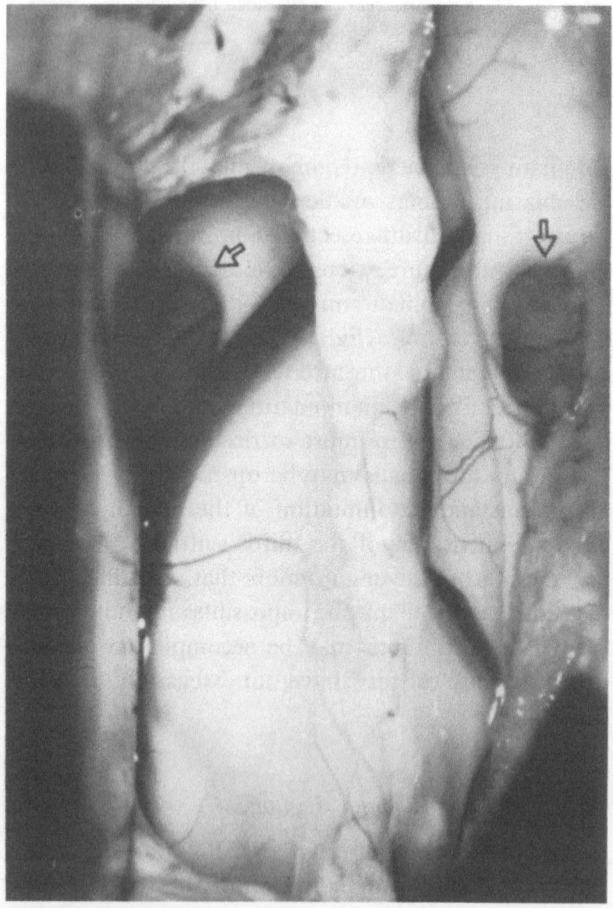

Fig. 3B. Operative photograph of transcallosal exposure showing both lateral ventricles and both foramina of Monro (arrows). A large colloid cyst is visible through the foramina of Monro

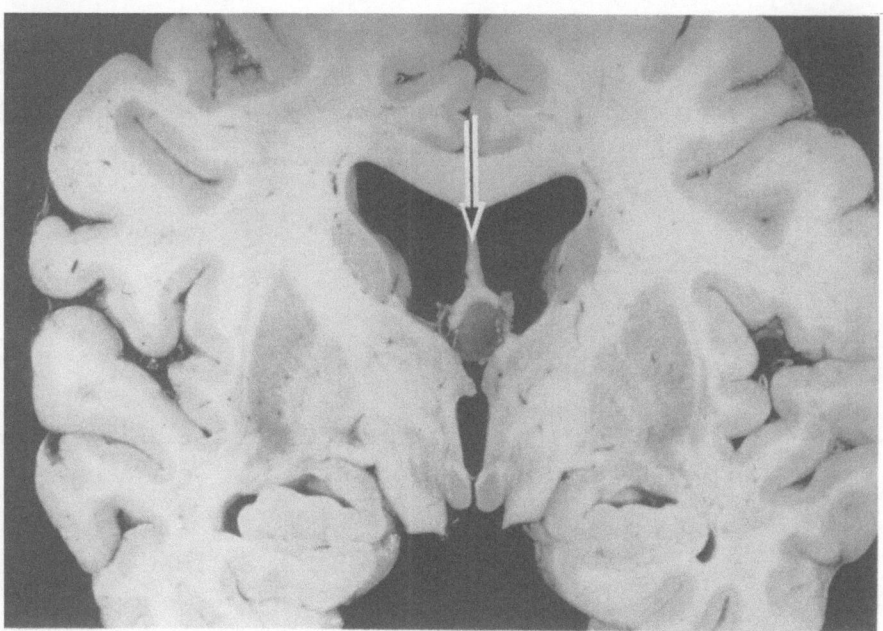

Fig. 3C. Coronal section of autopsy specimen of an incidental colloid cyst. The trajectory of the transcallosal exposure is indicated by an arrow emphasizing the direct approach to this lesion via the transcallosal route

the foramen of Monro is opened adequately, tumors may be removed by the standard microsurgical techniques of decompression and dissection around the capsule. Tumors most commonly encountered in this location are: astrocytoma, colloid cyst (Fig. 3), ependymoma, and craniopharyngioma. It should be remembered that craniopharyngiomas can arise from the floor of the third ventricle and grow to occupy the interior of this ventricle. Especially, in the example of the colloid cyst, the attachment will be at the posterior margin of the foramen of Monro.

(C) Posterior Third Ventricular Region

For tumors that occupy the posterior third ventricle (Fig. 4), there are a number of approaches that can be utilized. The critical issue to be discussed here is not the approach, but the location and size of the tumor as recognized on CT and NMR scans. The most common origin for tumors of this region is the pineal. However, other tumors may also arise from the thalamus (pulvinar) or the midbrain.

Those tumors which are eccentric and for the most part grow dorsal and lateral are exposed best by a lateral and not a midline exposure. In the case of thalamic (pulvinar) tumors a parafalx route, ipsilateral to the tumor, is preferred.

Turning to those midline tumors arising in the pineal, a variety of exposures have been recommended[11,14]. The most popular are: 1) Supratentorial occipital approach whereby the occipital lobe is retracted laterally or upward, the tentorium cut and

dissection carried out around the deep veins. 2) Posterior fossa infratentorial supracerebellar route (the one prefer[14]). This approach has the following advantages:

1) a midline exposure for midline tumors;
2) avoidance of injury to the parietal or occipital lobes;
3) entry to the tumor below the deep venous system[9].

The operation for the posterior fossa exposure is done in the sitting position with the patient's head fixated and flexed so that the tentorium is horizontal. A modest posterior fossa craniectomy is performed. This should extend lateral as far as possible and dorsal to include the torcular and transverse sinuses. It is not necessary to carry the craniectomy to the foramen magnum. The dura is opened widely to expose the dorsal surface of the cerebellum and the bridging veins are coagulated and divided. Two retractors are sufficient—one slightly elevating the tentorium and the other gently depressing the cerebellum (Fig. 5). If retraction of the cerebellum is considered suboptimal, dehydrating agents may be given. It is absolutely essential that the ventricular system be decompressed before the operative procedure and that, upon posterior fossa exposure, CSF is released from the cisterna magna. After the retractors are placed, the operation microscope is brought into position. It is arranged in the following manner. The oculars are angled upward to permit visibility in a comfortable position. The 250 or 275 mm objective is utilized. A self-retaining retractor system is conveniently arrayed around the operative incision so that the two aforementioned retractors may

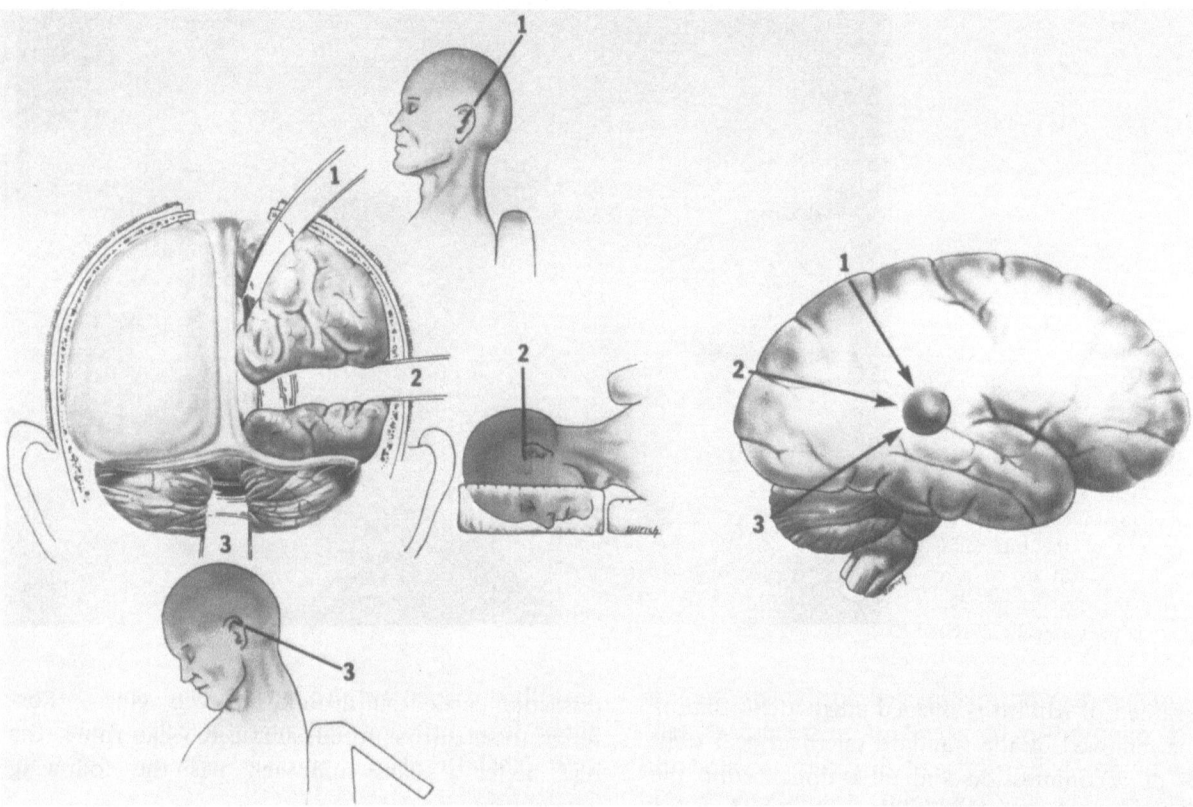

Fig. 4. Drawing indicating the various routes to the pineal region. The route illustrated in *1* is the classic parafalx route of Dandy. The route indicated in exposure *2* is that popularized by Poppen and Horrax. The route demonstrated in illustration *3* is that of Krausse, now utilized by Stein, which is the supracerebellar infratentorial approach

be positioned and locked. Additional arms are utilized for a tray containing cottonoids, a fixed irrigating system and a holder for various instruments. It is also essential that an adequate armrest be provided for the surgeon. With the operation microscope in position, the area of the incisura is visualized. The arachnoid over this area is always thickened in the presence of a tumor. This arachnoid is opened by sharp dissection and the following structures should be visualized: the vein of Galen, internal cerebral veins, veins of Rosenthal, and the precentral cerebellar vein. The posterior choroidal arteries are often displaced by the tumor and, except for their course over the capsule of the tumor, not visualized. In similar fashion, the deep venous system may be totally or partially obscured by the tumor. Normally, the deep venous system is adherent to or involved by the dorsal aspect of the tumor[9]. The cerebellum, once the arachnoid is divided, can be retracted away from the margin of the tumor exposing a maximal area of the posterior surface of the tumor (Fig. 6). Depending upon the consistency and density of the tumor various instruments may be utilized to form an internal decompression of the tumor. If the tumor is

soft and gelantinous a 5 or 7 Fr. suction tip may be utilized. For tumors which are firm, calcified or contain cartilage and muscle as well as bone, heavier instrumentation is needed including currettes, tumor forceps and an ultrasonic aspirator. We have found the long curved tip of the aspirator most useful in removing tumors of firm consistency. After performing an internal decompression, if the tumor is encapsulated and benign, the capsule is gently dissected away from the surrounding structures using microcautery, scissors and other microinstrumentation. If the tumor is malignant and invades the surrounding structures no attempt is made to totally remove it, but rather a generous internal decompression should be performed.

In our experience, it has been possible to remove approximately 30 percent of the tumors encountered in this region by techniques similar to those just described. The other 70% of tumors may be partly removed and decompressed. Following the tumor surgery, the closure is routine usually with partial or complete closure of the dura and then closure of the midline incision with drainage.

In discussing the surgical approach to posterior

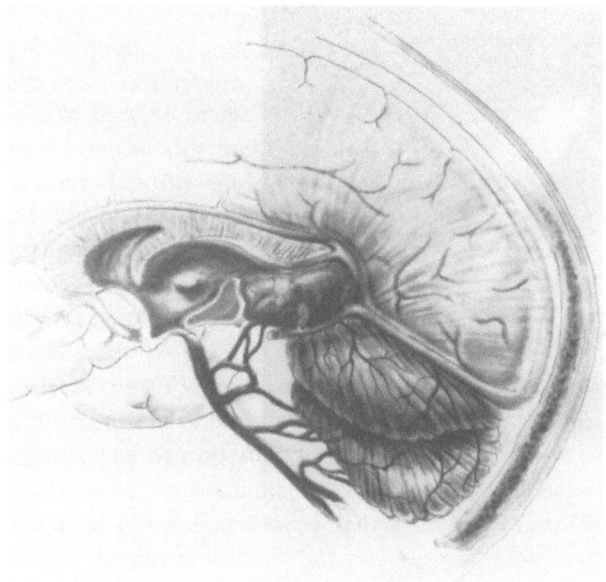

Fig. 5A. Sagittal drawing of a pineal tumor indicating the relationship to the surrounding structures

category includes the very benign teratoma which is well encapsulated and usually contains the three embryonal layers—in some cases two layers dermoids and epidermoids are also included in this category. These three types of tumors comprise the most benign germ cell tumors and are potentially resectable. At the other end of the spectrum are the malignant germ cell tumors including the germinoma composed of two definitive cell groups and similar histologically to the seminoma of the testicle or dysgerminoma of the ovary[1,7]. Germinomas can be cystic, tend to be invasive, but may have encapsulated portions. They have a propensity for metastasizing throughout the CSF spaces. Also included in the malignant variety of germ cell tumors are the highly malignant embryonal carcinoma. choriocarcinoma and various combinations of these tumors. The latter group are also invasive and can metastasize throughout the CSF spaces. We have found in recent cases a mixture of tumor types within a category. For example, we now have observed four patients who have

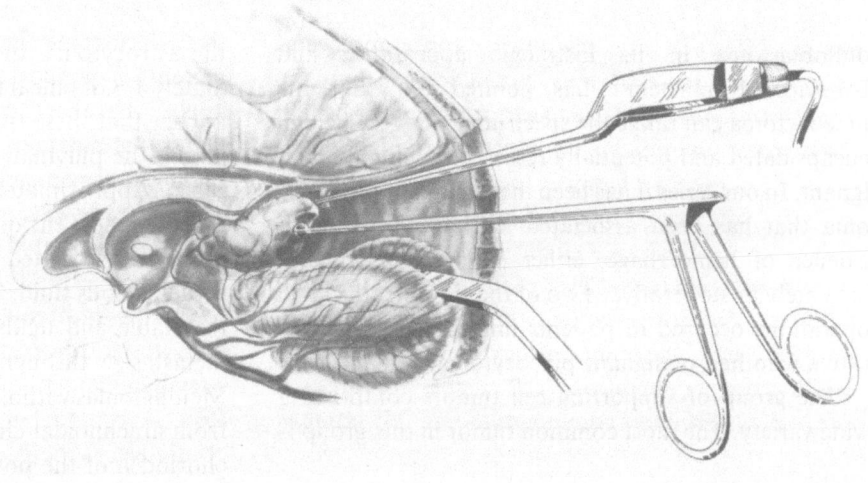

Fig. 5B. Sagittal drawing of the posterior fossa approach to a pineal tumor showing the positioning of a retractor and instruments

third ventricular or pineal region tumors, it is important to consider a scheme of histological identification for these tumors (Table 1).

With minor modifications we have categorized these tumors according to the scheme proposed by Herrick and Rubinstein[6,13]. The tumors are divided into three categories 1) germ cell origin tumors, 2) tumors arising from the pineal cells, 3) tumors arising from cells in surrounding or supporting structures related to the pineal. In each division there is a variety of tumors with a spectrum of benign to malignant types. The germ cell

teratomas in which approximately 90 to 95 percent of the volume of the tumor has been benign, but a small patch of five to ten percent of the volume is a malignant variety of tumor including germinoma, choriocarcinoma, or embryonal carcinoma mixed in with the benign elements. In these rare tumors the malignant area, although small, dictates the future course of growth and behavior of the tumor.

In those tumors which arise from pineal cells, there are two basic varieties, the pineocytoma and the pineoblastoma. The pineoblastoma resembles the me-

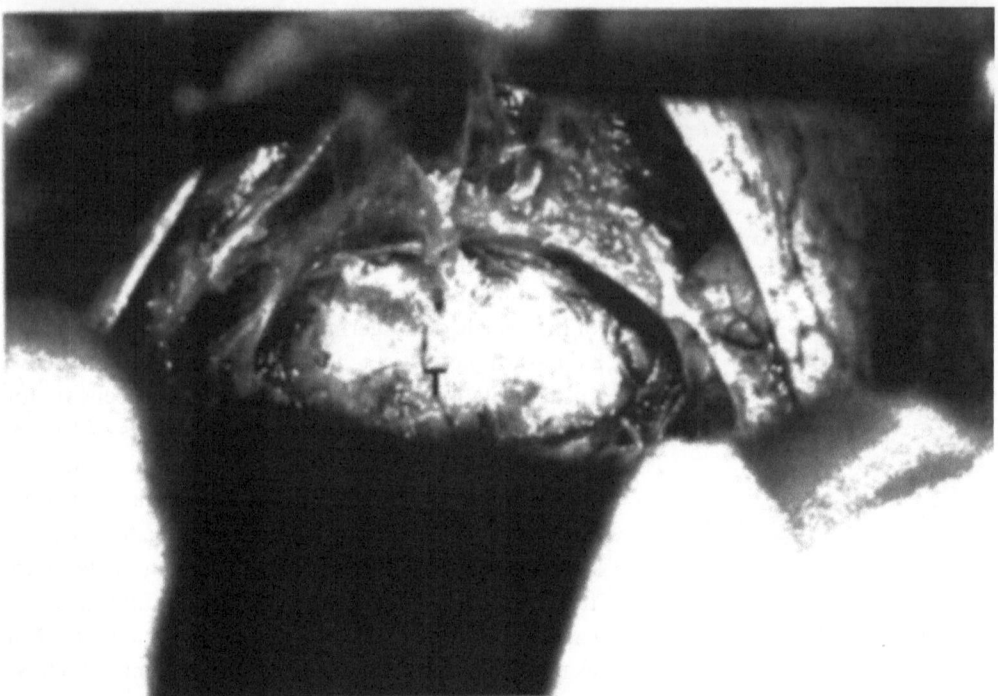

Fig. 6. Operative photograph of the incisural region showing an exposure of the posterior surface of a pineal tumor (*T*), which was a meningioma without dural attachment. The cerebellum lies in the foreground inferiorly and a retractor elevating the tentorium is superior

dulloblastoma in its histologic appearance and behavior. Rubinstein[13] has pointed out that the pineocytoma can range the spectrum from very benign encapsulated and potentially resectable to highly malignant. In our series it has been the malignant pineocytoma that has been associated with the greatest incidence of hemorrhage, either spontaneous or immediately postoperative. Two of the three deaths in 80 operations occured in patients immediately postoperative who had malignant pineocytomas.

The group of supporting cell tumors comprises a wide variety. The most common tumor in this group is the astrocytoma, including all four grades. Approximately 1/3 of pineal tumors are astrocytomas. It would appear that these tumors arise from within the pineal gland, the pulvinar region or the tectum of the midbrain. Approximately 50 percent of the astrocytomas are low grade, encapsulated and potentially resectable. Some are associated with large cysts containing yellow, proteinacious fluid. The malignant astrocytoma is not resectable and tends to invade locally, but does not metastasize throughout the central nervous system. Meningiomas without dural attachment appear to arise from arachnoidal cluster cells associated with the tela choriodea of the posterior roof of the third ventricle, intimate to the pineal gland[12]. These meningiomas are not rare and comprise six cases out of 80 pineal region tumors in our series. They are encapsulated, may attain large size and are potentially resectable. These meningiomas should be distinguished from the tentorial meningiomas which arise from the dura of the falx or tentorium. In the latter instance, the tumor is often dorsal to the internal cerebral veins and the vein of Galen. In the former instance of meningioma without dural attachment, the origin from the tela choroidea assures that the tumor will grow beneath the deep venous system and therefore displace it dorsally. The latter are best approached through the posterior fossa. Other tumor types falling into this group include

Table 1. *Classification of Pineal Tumors*

Germ cell origin	teratoma
	dermoid/epidermoid
	germinoma
	embryonal carcinoma
	choriocarcinoma
	mixed
Pineal cell origin	pineoblastoma
	pineocytoma
	benign
	malignant
Supporting cell origin	meningioma
	astrocytoma (all grades)
	ependymoma

ependymoma, oligodendroglioma, sarcoma and various other rare types.

The need to identify these tumors histologically is based on the aforementioned categorization. It is our premise that this wide variety of tumors can be treated effectively only if identified. The possible mixture of malignant and benign elements mandates that adequate biopsy or removal of the tumor be accomplished. It has been suggested that these tumors be identified by stereotactic biopsy currently carried out through the assist of the CT scan. In such instances, a small amount of tissue will be obtained. It may be difficult for even an experienced neuropathologist to make a diagnosis on the basis of this small amount of material. This is why we have not yet embraced the technique of needle biopsy for pineal tumors, but prefer open biopsy with resection or a generous internal decompression in most cases. In our experience, the neuroradiological diagnosis of pineal tumors, even assisted by an analysis of the biological markers, does not accurately diagnose the nature of these tumors. Our experience with NMR scanning is limited and perhaps when this comes into wider use, we will be able to diagnose these tumors with greater accuracy in lieu of histological confirmation.

With the histological diagnosis, we have a foundation for subsequent therapy. For the group of 30 percent of the lesions which are benign and encapsulated, surgical resection is the treatment of choice. For the germinomas, comprising approximately 30 percent of tumors, we advocate radiotherapy as the primary treatment[10,14,17]. Postoperatively the lumbar spinal fluid is evaluated three times for cytology and regardless of these findings, a myelogram is performed[5]. If there is no evidence of tumor metastases to the spinal region, then radiation is concentrated on the pineal tumor and the third ventricular area with 5,000 rads and a lesser dose in the range of 3,500 rads to the rest of the brain. If the spine is involved then 3,500 rads are given in this area. If these tumors have recurred after treatment with radiotherapy, then we have used the chemotherapeutic regime after Einhorn, consisting of cis-platinum, vinblastine and bleomycin[2,4]. In the astrocytomas which comprise approximately 30 percent of the tumors of this region, total removal may be carried out; if it cannot, local radiotherapy is given. The embryonal carcinoma, choriocarcinoma and other tumors of this primitive series are treated primarily by chemotherapy[8]. Radiotherapy has not been used in conjunction with chemotherapy in these tumors and our experience is too limited to make any prediction for the future course of combined therapy. The pineoblastoma and malignant pineocytoma are treated by radiotherapy.

References

1. Anderson, T., Waldman, T. A., Javadpour, N., et al., NIH conference: testicular germ cell neoplasms: recent advances in diagnosis and therapy. Ann. Int. Med. 90 (1979), 373–385.
2. Allen, J. C., Helson, L., High-dose cyclophosphamide chemotherapy for recurrent CNS tumors in children. J. Neurosurg. 44 (1981), 749–756.
3. DeGirolami, U., Schmidek, H., Clinicopathological study of 53 tumors of the pineal region. J. Neurosurg. 39 (1973), 455–462.
4. Einhorn, L. H., Donohue, J., Cis-diamine dichloroplatinum, vinblastine, and bleomycin combination chemotherapy in disseminated testicular cancer. Ann. Int. Med. 87 (1977), 293–298.
5. Gindhart, T. D., Tsukahara, Y. C., Cytologic diagnosis of pineal germinoma in cerebrospinal fluid and sputum. Acta Cytologica 23 (1979), 341–346.
6. Herrick, M. K., Rubinstein, L. J., The cytological differentiating potential of pineal parenchymal neoplasms (the pinealomas). A clinicopathological study of 28 tumors. Brain 102 (1979), 321–332.
7. Neuwelt, E. A., Ginsberg, M., Frenkel, et al., Malignant pineal region tumors: A clinico-pathological study. J. Neurosurg. 57 (1979), 597–607.
8. Ono, N., Takeda, F, Uki, J., et al., A supracellar embryonal carcinoma producing alphafetoprotein and human chorionic gonadotropin; treated with combined chemotherapy followed by radiotherapy. Surg. Neurol. 18 (1983), 435–443.
9. Quest, D. O., Kleriga, E., Microsurgical anatomy of the pineal region. Neurosurg. 6 (1979), 385–390.
10. Rao, Y. T. R., Medini, E., Haselow R. E., et al., Pineal and ectopic pineal tumors: the role of radiation therapy. Cancer 48 (1981), 708–713.
11. Reid, W. S., Clark, K., Comparison of the infratentorial and transtentorial approaches to the pineal region. Neurosurg. 3 (1978), 1–8.
12. Rozario, R., Adelman, L., Prager, R. J., Stein, B. M., Meningiomas of the pineal region and third ventricle. Neurosurg. 5 (1979), 489–495.
13. Rubinstein, L. F., Cytogenesis and differentiation of pineal neoplasms. Hum. Path. 12 (1981), 441–448.
14. Stein, B. M., Supracerebellar approach for pineal region neoplasms. Operative Neurosurgical Techniques, Vol. 1 (Schmidek, H., Sweet, W., eds.), pp. 599–607. Grune & Stratton. 1982.
15. Stein, B. M., Third ventricular tumors. Clin. Neurosurg. Chap.17, Vol. 27, pp. 315–331. P. W. Carmel. 1981.
16. Stein, B. M., Fraser, R. A. R., Tenner, M.S., Third ventricular tumors in children. J. Neurol. Neurosurg. Psychiat. 35 (1972), 776–778.
17. Sung, D., Harisiadis, L., Chang, C. H., Midline pineal tumors and suprasellar germinomas: highly curable by irradiation. Radiology 128 (1978), 745–751.

Author's address: Benett M. Stein, M.D., Professor of Neurosurgery, Neurological Institute of New York, Department of Neurosurgery, College of Physicians and Surgeons of Columbia University, 710 West 168th Street, New York, NY 10032, U.S.A.

Acta Neurochirurgica, Suppl. 35, 50–54 (1985)

Approaches to the Pineal Region

G. Pendl

Department of Neurosurgery, University of Vienna Medical School, Wien, Austria

Summary

On the basis of anatomical studies in fresh cadavers, formalin fixed brains and clinical experiences in 40 surgically treated cases of pineal and midbrain lesions the most important surgical approaches with their anatomical peculiarities as well as pitfalls are demonstrated. Emphasis is given to the great vein of Galen and its tributaries as major obstacle in microsurgery in this area.

Keywords: Microsurgical anatomy; pineal region; surgical approaches.

Introduction

Surgery of the pineal region in the past was not very encouraging. Lesions of the pineal gland and those arising from the environs of the pineal region and involving the posterior third ventricle as well as the quadrigeminal plate are deep-seated in the center of the head. Surgical removal of these lesions was and still is considered to be both dangerous and tedious with mortality rates of no less than 50% (Pia 1954) in the past.

But since microneurosurgical techniques have eliminated many hazards in this central-most part of the brain and the anatomy of this region has become better understood a more rational surgical approach to this region emerged (Pendl 1984, 1985, Quest *et al.* 1980, Rhoton *et al.* 1981, Yamamoto *et al.* 1981). Various surgical approaches were developed in the past and the purpose of this investigation is to point out their pitfalls especially in regard of the great vein of Galen and its tributaries.

Material and Methods

This study is based on the results obtained in 26 cadaver brains studied under microsurgical operating conditions as well as 6 human brains fixed in formalin, whose vascular systems were previously injected with acrylates. The findings were compared with the surgical exposures and the personal experience in 40 pineal region lesions, with intrinsic midbrain lesions in 15, and with surgery related mortality in 3 (7.5%).

Observations and Discussion

On the basis of clinical and morphological findings the pineal gland tumors and those of the posterior part of the third ventricle as well as various other lesions of the quadrigeminal cistern like arachnoid cysts, meningiomas and vein of Galen aneurysm, are grouped together as pineal lesions necessitating attention to the same anatomical structures, especially the tributaries of the vein of Galen, when surgically approached. The different approaches to this region recommended in the literature (Pendl 1984) are greatly influenced by the deep veins rather than by the arteries: their course determines the choice of the operative approach.

Fig. 1 shows the common course of the arteries and veins schematically. The deep venous structures of the vein of Galen and its tributaries form a roof-like dense venous network above the pineal gland and the quadrigeminal plate (Fig. 2). Their vulnerability was the main cause of the pessimistic attitude towards surgery of pineal region lesions.

Fig. 3 demonstrates the 4 most important and established approaches to the pineal-midbrain region. The historical perspectives of pineal lesion surgery is important for the efforts; for the ongoing discussion of what access to choose, see elsewhere (Pendl 1984, Zülch 1981). Since the various surgical approaches reported in the literature incorporates many personal and individualistic characteristics developed mainly by macrosurgical techniques, they should be compared and

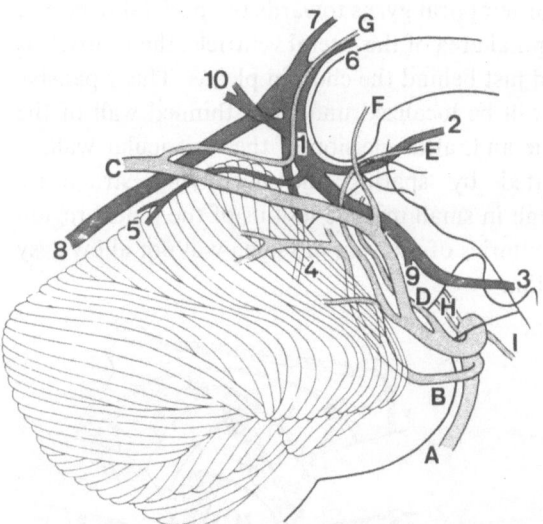

Fig. 1. Schematic representation of the arteries and veins of the midbrain and pineal region. *A* basilar artery; *B* superior cerebellar artery; *C* posterior cerebral artery; *D* common trunc of the quadrigeminal and geniculate body artery; *E* median posterior choroidal artery; *F* lateral posterior choroidal artery; *G* posterior pericallosal artery; *H* posterior thalmoperforating arteries; *1* great vein of Galen; *2* internal cerebral vein; *3* basal vein of Rosenthal; *4* precentral cerebellar vein; *5* superior vermian vein; *6* posterior pericallosal vein; *7* inferior sagittal sinus; *8* straight sinus; *9* mesencephalic vein; *10* internal occipital vein

1. Transcallosal Approach

Originally described by Dandy in 1921, this approach was preferred by most neurosurgeons in the pre-microsurgical era, although it was associated with a high mortality rate of up to 90%, which could be reduced by modern neurosurgical equipment from 67% to 4% (Hoffman 1984). Fig. 4 demonstrates the exposure of a pineal lesion by this approach in a schematic drawing showing how the deep veins block the access both to pineal tumors and, even more so, to the quadrigeminal cistern and plate in midbrain tumors. The site and length of the craniotomy in the parieto-occipital region parallel to the sagittal sinus depend on the location of the major bridging veins to the sinus in the angiogram. The dura mater is flapped towards the sinus, evacuation of CSF from hydrocephally enlarged ventricles helps to retract the parieto-occipital lobe between draining veins from the falx in order to expose the splenium of the corpus callosum, which has to be transected for 1–2 cm, depending on the extension of the lesion. It may also be necessary to incise the inferior sagittal sinus vertically and the lower part of the falx in order to obtain a better view of the

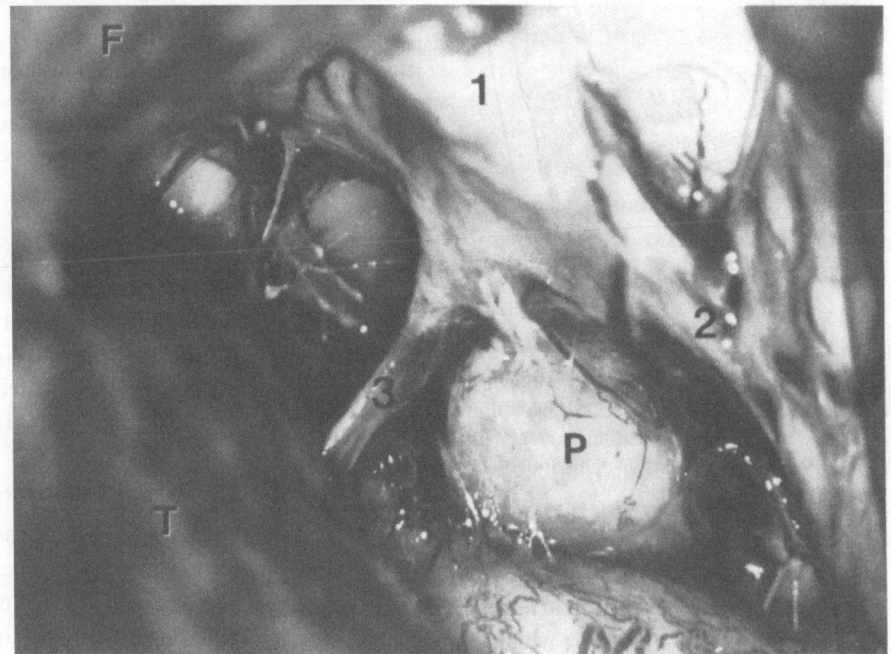

Fig. 2. Oblique view from right-occipital into the quadrigeminal cistern in a fresh cadaver. *P* pineal gland; *F* falx; *T* tentorium; *1* great vein of Galen; *2* right basal vein of Rosenthal; *3* precentral cerebellar vein

reevaluated versus microsurgical techniques. We will confine our study to the 4 most important approaches:

1. Transcallosal,
2. transventricular,
3. occipital transtentorial,
4. infratentorial supracerebellar.

opposite side. The vein of Galen with both the internal cerebral veins and the basal veins of Rosenthal as well as the medial occipital vein prevent access to moderately sized pineal tumors and even more so, to the quadrigeminal plate or ambient cistern. Therefore, we consider this approach to the pineal region and midbrain the least feasible, except in vein of Galen

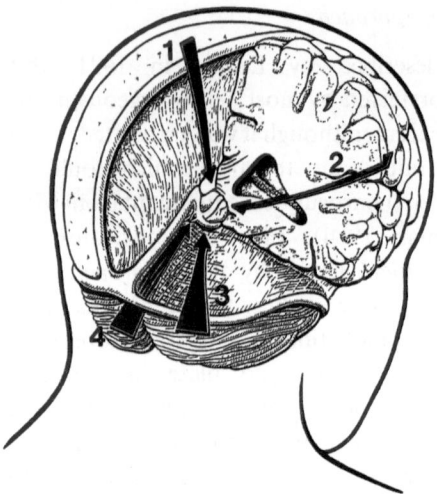

Fig. 3. Schematic demonstration of the 4 most important approaches to the pineal region. *1* transcallosal approach; *2* transventricular approach; *3* occipital transtentorial approach; *4* infratentorial supracerebellar approach

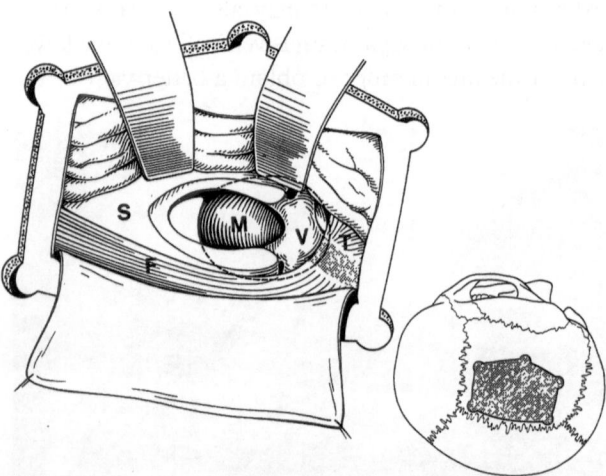

Fig. 4. Transcallosal approach with position of the head with site of craniotomy in accordance with the schematic drawing of the exposure of a mass lesion. *M* mass lesion; *V* great vein of Galen with its tributaries; *S* corpus callosum with transsected splenium; *F* falx; *T* tentorium

aneurysms where the feeding arteries are best exposed by this approach or in tumors which expand anteriorly into the third ventricle and those extending upward into the corpus callosum (Hoffman 1984).

2. Transventricular Approach

This approach, published by Van Wagenen in 1931, uses the hydrocephalically enlarged lateral ventricles for access. After an L-shaped cortical incision in the

superior temporal gyrus towards the parietal region of the trigonal area of the lateral ventricle, the ventricle is reached just behind the choroid plexus. The expansive lesion will be localized under the thinned wall of the ventricle and, after incision of the ventricular wall, is enucleated by sparing the deep-lying structures. Although in small midline lesions of the pineal region the tributaries of the vein of Galen will not allow easy dissection.

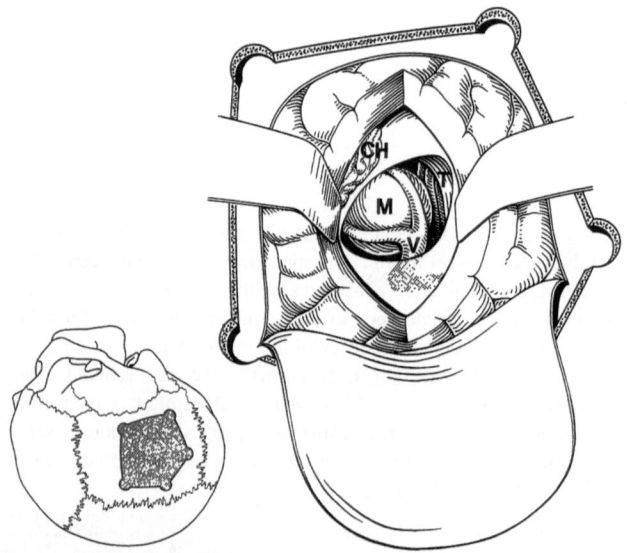

Fig. 5. Transventricular approach with position of the head with site of craniotomy in accordance with the schematic drawing of the exposure of a mass lesion. *M* mass lesion; *V* great vein of Galen with its tributaries; *T* tentorium; *CH* choroidal plexus of the right lateral ventricle

Fig. 5 schematically shows the exposure of the pineal lesion by a transventricular approach with the vein of Galen and the basal vein of Rosenthal obstructing access; the variable internal occipital vein is not included in the drawing. This approach should be confined to lesions extending more laterally to one side.

3. Occipital Transtentorial Approach

This approach described by Heppner in 1959 was popularized by Poppen (1966), although his version is far too narrow and technically difficult, therefore the modification of Jamieson (1971) is preferred by most surgeons (Neuwelt and Batjer 1984). In this approach the patient is usually placed in a semisitting position and the craniotomy is made close to the sagittal and right transverse sinuses over the occipital pole. The dura mater is incised in a T-shaped or stellate fashion and the occipital lobe is retracted superiorly and laterally. Bridging veins have to be sacrificed, occasionally also those from the inferior aspect of the occipital

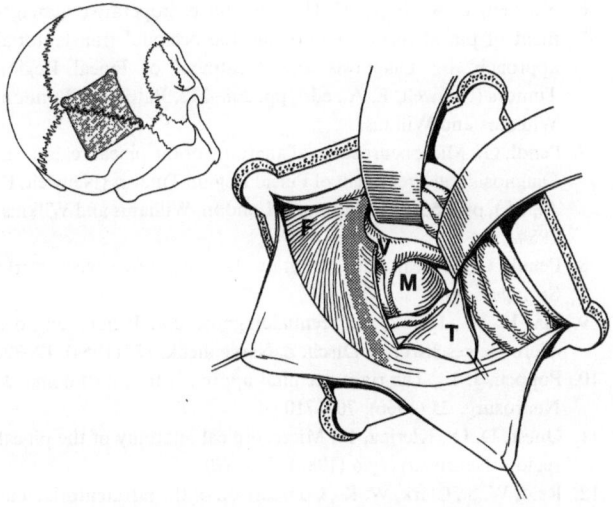

Fig. 6. Occipital transtentorial approach with position of the head with site of craniotomy in accordance with the schematic drawing of the exposure of a mass lesion. *M* mass lesion; *V* great vein of Galen with its tributaries; *F* falx; *T* tentorium, incised.

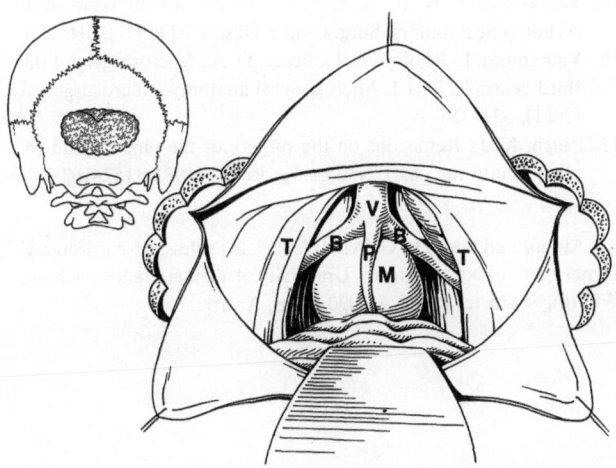

Fig. 7. Infratentorial supracerebellar approach with position of the head and site of craniectomy in accordance with the schematic drawing of the exposure of a mass lesion. *M* mass lesion; *V* great vein of Galen; *P* precentral cerebellar vein; *B* basal vein of Rosenthal; *T* tentorium

lobe to the transverse sinus and tentorium. When the tentorial edge is reached it is incised parallel to the straight sinus and both edges are retracted with sutures to expose the arachnoid folds of the quadrigeminal cistern, if not the lesion itself. A good view of the splenium with the Galenic venous system and of the quadrigeminal plate is provided. Care has to be taken not to injure the posterior cerebral artery with the calcarine fissure and the internal occipital vein by retraction, while the precentral cerebellar vein can be sacrificed without any unfavourable results. Fig. 6 schematically demonstrates the exposure of a pineal lesion by this approach with the roof-like venous structure on top of the lesion excluding the precentral cerebellar vein. Reid and Clark (1978) compared this approach to the infratentorial approach; they believe that the occipital transtentorial approach gives a broader range of exposure and have also used it for vein of Galen aneurysms.

4. Infratentorial Supracerebellar Approach

Special credit must be given to Stein (1971) for reviving this surgical approach to the pineal region which was first described by Krause in 1911. In this approach, a suboccipital craniotomy with exposure of the torcula and extension well above the transverse sinus bilaterally to allow upward retraction of the tentorium, if necessary, is performed with the patient usually in a sitting position. It is possible to spare the arch of atlas and the foramen. After the dura is opened by a Y-shaped cut and bridging veins from the cerebellar hemispheres and vermis to the tentorium are sacrificed, the cerebellum sinks down and leaves a wide enough gap under the tentorium to the quadrigeminal cistern. Almost no further dislocation downward with a retractor is necessary. The dense opalescent arachnoid folds of the quadrigeminal cistern obstruct the topography of the quadrigeminal cistern and must be divided by sharp dissection in order not to tear the vascular structures. After dissection, the quadrigeminal plate with the pineal gland and veins is sufficiently well exposed. The roof-like deeper venous structures are equally well exposed above the operative field; occasionally, only the precentral cerebellar vein must be sacrificed without any adverse effects. Removal of a lesion in the pineal region usually leaves a large opening to the posterior third ventricle. On the lateral aspects of the quadrigeminal cistern small branches of the median posterior choroidal artery are encountered and may be sacrificed without adverse effects. Fig. 7 shows this approach schematically in a pineal mass lesion.

In order to expose the quadrigeminal plate and reach the ambient cistern the anterior margin of the cerebellar hemisphere close to the vermis has to be incised for 1 or 2 cm.

Conclusion

The feasibility for a direct surgical attack upon lesions of the pineal and midbrain regions is dependent on the angioarchitecture of the pineal region. Most important for the approach to choose is the course of the vein of Galen and its tributaries. Therefore, the infratentorial approach is recommended; an alternative route is the occipital transtentorial approach. Both adequately protect the deep veins and help to explore the pineal region in all respects. Either approach provides a safe adequate exposure to the pineal region. The transcallosal approach is considered as the most inadequate, although it was preferred for many years, because it is associated with greater surgical risks. Lesions extending or arising more laterally may be better approached by a transventricular route. Microtopographic studies and the surgical experience in the past 12 years seem to support this attitude.

References

1. Dandy, W. E., An operation for the removal of pineal tumors. Surg. Gynec. Obstet. *33* (1921), 113–119.
2. Heppner, F., Zur operativen Technik bei Pinealomen. Zbl. Neurochir. *19* (1959), 219–224.
3. Hoffman, H. J., Transcallosal approach to pineal tumors and the Hospital for Sick Children Series of pineal region tumors. In: Diagnosis and Treatment of Pineal Region Tumors (Neuwelt, E.A., ed.), pp. 223–235. Baltimore-London: Williams and Wilkins. 1984.
4. Jamieson, K. G., Excision of pineal tumors. J. Neurosurg. *35* (1971), 550–553.
5. Krause, F., Chirurgie des Gehirns und Rückenmarks, Bd. 1. Berlin-Wien: Urban und Schwarzenberg. 1911.
6. Neuwelt, E. A., Bajer, H. H., Pre- and postoperative management of pineal region tumors and the occipital transtentorial approach. In: Diagnosis and Treatment of Pineal Region Tumors (Neuwelt, E. A., ed.), pp. 208–222. Baltimore-London: Williams and Wilkins.
7. Pendl, G., Microneurosurgical anatomy of the pineal region. In: Diagnosis and Treatment of Pineal Region Tumors (Neuwelt, E. A., ed.), pp. 155–207. Baltimore-London: Williams and Wilkins. 1984.
8. Pendl, G., Pineal and Midbrain Lesions. Wien-New York: Springer. 1985.
9. Pia, H. W., Klinik, Differentialdiagnose und Behandlung der Vierhügelgeschwülste. Dtsch. Z. Nervenheilk. *172* (1954), 12–32.
10. Poppen, J. L., The right occipital approach to a pinealoma. J. Neurosurg. *25* (1966), 706–710.
11. Quest, D. O., Kleriga, E., Microsurgical anatomy of the pineal region. Neurosurgery *6* (1980), 385–390.
12. Reid, W. S., Clark, W. K., Comparison of the infratentorial and transtentorial approaches to the pineal region. Neurosurgery *3* (1978), 1–8.
13. Rhoton, A. L., Yamamoto, I., Peace, D. A., Microsurgery of the third ventricle: Part 2. Operative approaches. Neurosurgery *8* (1981), 357–373.
14. Stein, B. M., The infratentorial supracerebellar approach to pineal lesions. J. Neurosurg. *35* (1971), 197–202.
15. Van Wagenen, W. P., A surgical approach for the removal of certain pineal tumors. Surg. Gynec. Obstet. *53* (1931), 216–220.
16. Yamamoto, I., Rhoton, A. L., Peace, D. A., Microsurgery of the third ventricle: Part 1. Microsurgical anatomy. Neurosurgery *8* (1981), 334–356.
17. Zülch, K. J., Reflexions on the surgery of the pineal gland (A glimpse into the past). Neurosurg. Rev. *4* (1981), 152–162.

Author's address: Dr. G. Pendl, Associate Professor Neusorurgery, Department of Neurosurgery, University of Vienna Medical School, Währinger Gürtel 18-20, A-1090 Wien, Austria.

Acta Neurochirurgica, Suppl. 35, 55–59 (1985)

E. Diagnosis

Diagnosis of Lesions in the Third Ventricle

E. Schindler

Department of Neurosurgery, University of Vienna Medical School, Wien, Austria

Summary

The precise diagnosis of lesions occupying the third ventricle requires both clinical and radiological examinations. Laboratory tests may provide important additional information in some cases. The specific diagnosis of a third ventricle tumor, however, cannot be established without biopsy except in very rare cases. The diagnostic and differential diagnostic problems are illustrated by some examples and discussed.

Keywords: CT in third ventricle tumors; diagnostic methods in third ventricle tumors; germinoma; third ventricle tumors.

Precisely diagnosing a space-occupying lesion in the third ventricle requires attention to both clinical and radiological findings. The clinical examination has to be the first diagnostic step in each case, even though sophisticated neuroimaging techniques are available. While clinical signs and symptoms may be suggestive of such a tumor, they do not provide definite evidence. Focal signs pointing to an involvement of central cerebral structures—if present at all—are often disguised by unspecific symptoms of increased intracranial pressure. On the other hand, such focal signs are not necessarily due to a midline tumor. Parinaud's syndrome is not always caused by a midbrain tumor but may be due to a vascular disorder, to stenosis of the Sylvian aqueduct, a space-occupying lesion of a cerebral hemisphere, or even to subdural hematoma[8, 14, 18]. Furthermore, endocrine disorders without any neurological deficit[21] may occur in third ventricle tumors and misdirect diagnostic attention.

Thus, whenever a space-occupying lesion in the third ventricle is suspected, radiological examinations must be done to get the essential information for adequate therapy and rational prognosis. The first step is to make sure whether there is really a tumor or not. If there is, its size and the involvement of adjacent structures have to be determined. But for planning adequate therapy more information is needed. It is important to know whether the tumor has invaded or is merely compressing the surrounding nervous tissue; whether it is benign or malignant and has seeded or not; it would be essential to know whether the tumor is sensitive to radiation or to cytostatic agents, particularly as progress in neurosurgery, radiotherapy and chemotherapy has improved the prognosis of third ventricle tumors.

Currently, the most useful method for diagnosing intracranial tumors is CT. With this examination a third ventricle tumor can either be detected or ruled out in nearly all cases, and the tumor size can be assessed as well as the involvement of adjacent structures. However, CT does not contribute information on tumor biology and histology. As for NMR, it has not yet been established whether or not it will provide unequivocal evidence of tumor histology.

Radiological findings and diagnostic problems in third ventricle tumors shall be illustrated by some examples. Fig. 1 shows a markedly enhanced tumor on the floor of the third ventricle with apparently sharply delineated margins. Based on the CT findings, expansive tumor growth was assumed. At surgery, however, an infiltrating tumor was found; thus, total removal was ruled out. The histological diagnosis was malignant teratoma.

In another case CT (Fig. 2a) suggested a pineal region tumor invading cerebral structures. The lesion was thought to be inoperable, and radiotherapy was initiated after shunting. This was wrong, since, a few

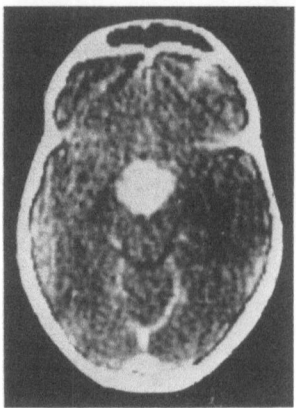

Fig. 1. CT after intravenous contrast. Tumor on the third ventricle floor with well delineated margins and marked homogeneous enhancement. (Histological diagnosis: malignant teratoma)

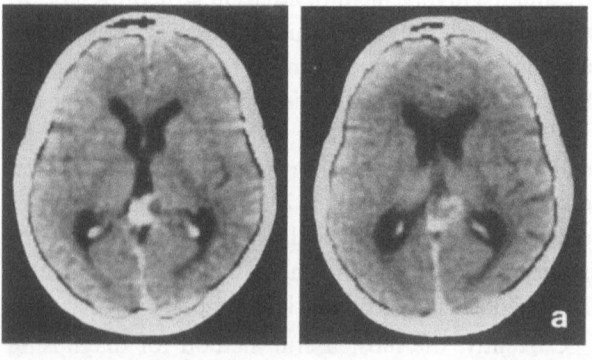

weeks later, angiography revealed an arteriovenous malformation involving the great vein of Galen (Fig. 2b). This case emphasizes once again that, in all midline lesions, angiography should be the next diagnostic step after CT. In particular, the location and the function of the deep venous system have to be assessed before operating on a third ventricle tumor. Thus, both carotid and vertebral angiographies are indicated in order to visualize all the vessels which may possibly be involved. Moreover, the specific diagnosis of the lesion can be established by angiography in some cases (Fig. 2b).

The CT findings shown in Fig. 3 are consistent with germinoma[6, 24, 26]: There is a well delineated homogeneously hyperdense mass without calcification on the third ventricle floor; tumor spread is present in both anterior horns; the tumor tissue shows marked and homogeneous enhancement, and in the enhanced scan an additional tumor in the pineal region is distinctly visualized (Fig. 3b). In this case the radiological diagnosis was double midline germinoma[20] with ventricular metastases. This was confirmed by CSF cytology, since germinoma cells were identified. CT signs of ventricular metastases are, however, not specific for germinoma—such metastases may also occur in other germ cell tumors, malignant gliomas, pineal parenchymal tumors, choroid plexus papillomas, ependymomas, medulloblastomas, and even in melanomas and malignant lymphomas[10, 12, 13]. Differential diagnostic information may be obtained by CSF examination[16, 21]. CSF

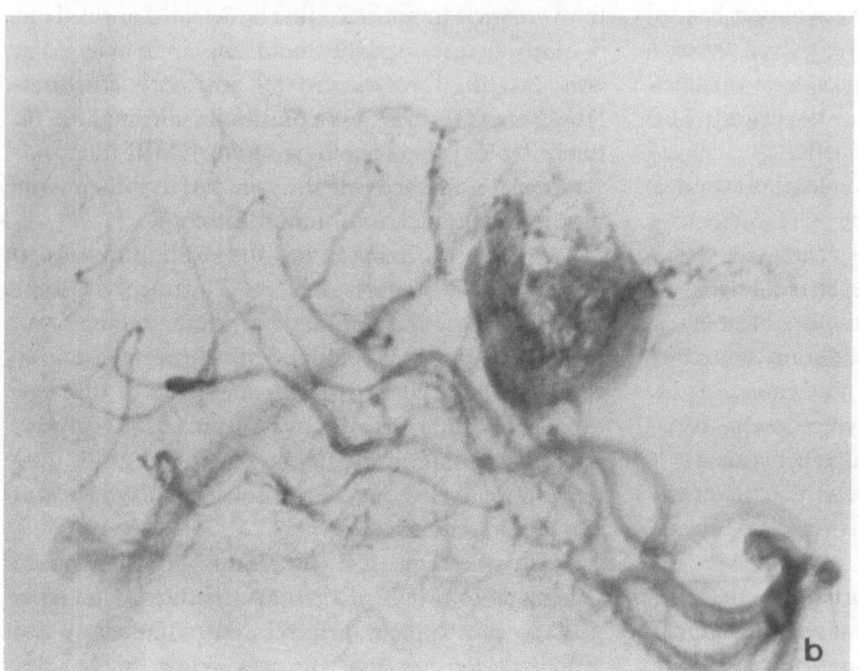

Fig. 2. a) CT after contrast: enhancing lesion in the pineal region involving the posterior portion of the third ventricle; slight ventricular dilatation; b) vertebral angiography: arteriovenous malformation involving the great vein of Galen

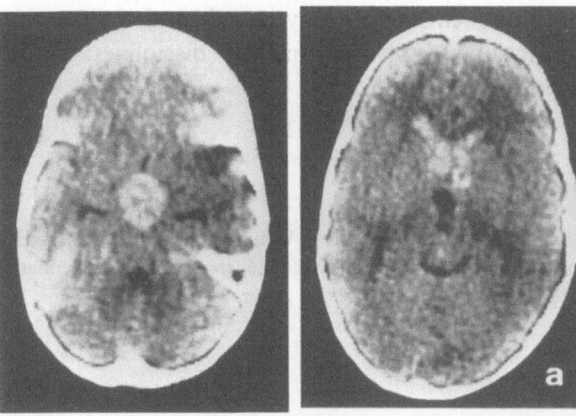
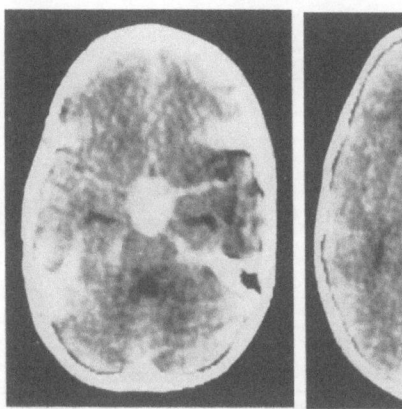
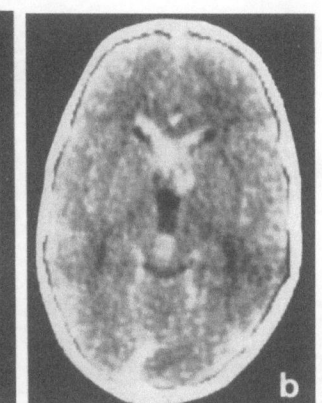

Fig. 3. a) Plain CT; b) CT after intravenous contrast. Homogeneously hyperdense tumors on the third ventricle floor and in the pineal region with tumor spread in both anterior horns; marked enhancement. (Radiological diagnosis: double midline germinoma)

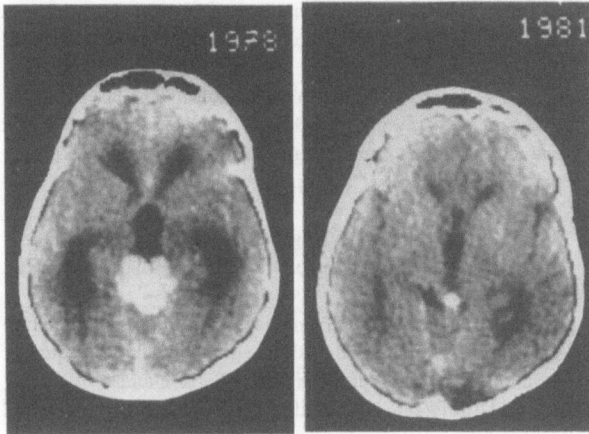

Fig. 4. Pineal region germinoma before and after treatment. Three years after radiotherapy no tumor is discernible. (Enhanced scans)

cytology, therefore, should be considered in all third ventricle tumors.

It is well known that germinomas are highly sensitive to radiation and may even be cured by radiotherapy[6, 7, 19, 23]. CT follow-up studies showed that intracranial germinomas may disappear after irradiation with no more than 20 to 30 Gy[6]. Fig. 4 shows the CT of a pineal region germinoma (verified by biopsy) before and after treatment—three years after radiotherapy no tumor is discernible, the patient is free from disease. In my opinion, this is one of the rare conditions that justify radiotherapy of an intracranial tumor without verification of its histology. This means that, if a homogeneous mass with well delineated margins and marked homogeneous enhancement is detected by CT (these findings are highly suggestive of germinoma), the tumor should be irradiated without operation. CT follow-up examinations during radiotherapy are, of course, imperative in such a case. On the other hand, if

the CT signs are not typical of germinoma, radiotherapy without histological verification will remain "a shot in the dark" as Cushing[4] has stated about half a century ago.

In most cases, however, the specific diagnosis of a third ventricle tumor cannot be established by CT or by other neuroradiological methods. Histologically identical tumors often do not show the same appearance on CT. Conversely, the CT scans of histologically different tumors may be very similar so that differentiation is not possible. In Fig. 5 as well as in Fig. 6 rather inhomogeneously enhancing tumors with irregular margins are seen—the tumor in Fig. 5 proved to be an ependymoma, that in Fig. 6 a pineoblastoma.

Considering the diagnostic problems in third ventricle tumors, one must be aware that, in many cases, not all the problems can be solved, in particular that information on tumor histology cannot be obtained without biopsy (except in very rare cases). However, if clinical as well as neuroradiological examinations and laboratory tests are performed, the greatest possible diagnostic accuracy can be achieved.

It goes without saying that neurological, ophthalmological and endocrinological examinations are imperative in every third ventricle tumor. Hormone studies are required to assess a possible involvement of the hypothalamus or the pituitary.

Plain films provide important information, particularly in children with increased intracranial pressure. The diagnostic value of CT and angiography is obvious. Ventriculography may be indicated in special cases, but is rather seldom needed since CT has become available. NMR will certainly prove to be very useful in diagnosing third ventricle tumors; at present, however, it seems to be rather a matter of research than a method that routinely solves diagnostic problems.

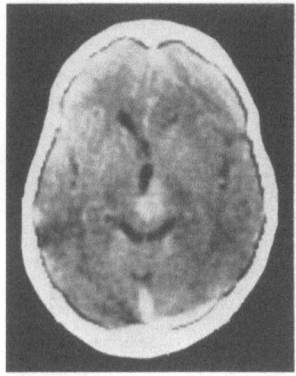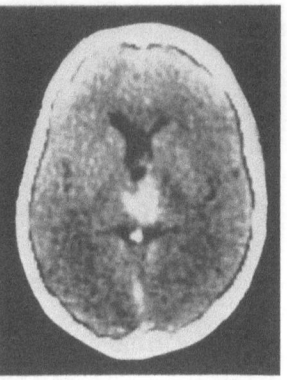

Fig. 5. CT after intravenous contrast. Tumor involving the posterior portion of the third ventricle and the pineal region. Slightly inhomogeneous enhancement, irregular tumor margins. (Histological diagnosis: ependymoma)

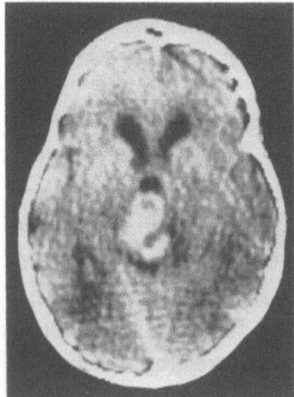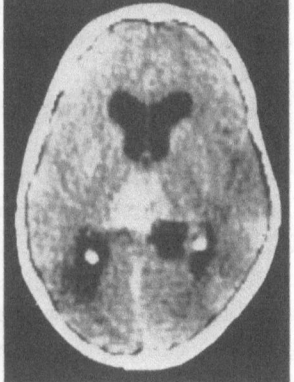

Fig. 6. CT after intravenous contrast. Tumor involving the third ventricle and the pineal region. Inhomogeneous enhancement, irregular tumor margins. (Histological diagnosis: pineoblastoma)

In some cases a specific diagnosis of a third ventricle tumor can be made by laboratory tests. This is possible when tumor cells are identified in the CSF. In very rare cases tumor markers reveal the histological diagnosis. Intracranial choriocarcinomas and yolk sac tumors are usually located in the midline and predominantly occur in young patients[5, 9, 15, 17, 22]. Therefore, analyses of human chorionic gonadotropin—to confirm or rule out choriocarcinoma—should be done in all children with third ventricle tumors[1,9,15], even if there are no signs of precocious puberty. Analyses of alphafetoprotein—a marker of yolk sac tumors—should be done as well[1,2,17, 25]. These analyses are also indicated for follow-ups after therapy[1, 2, 9, 15, 25]. The role of melatonin as a tumor marker of neoplasms originating from pineal cells[3, 11] is not yet clear, but it may become important as soon as pineal biology is better understood.

It is evident that progress in therapeutic methods is always a challenge to improve diagnostic accuracy.

This improvement can only be achieved by intensive cooperation of different medical disciplines; this is evident as well.

Acknowledgement

I am indebted to Prof. Dr. S. Wende, head of the Neuroradiological Department of the University Hospital of Mainz, Germany, for the illustrations shown in this paper.

References

1. Allen, J. C., Nisselbaum, J., Epstein, F., Rosen, G., Schwartz, M. K., Alphafetoprotein and human chorionic gonadotropin determination in cerebrospinal fluid. An aid to the diagnosis and management of intracranial germ-cell tumors. J. Neurosurg. 51 (1979), 368–374.
2. Arita, N., Bitoh, S., Ushio, Y., Hayakawa, T., Hasegawa, H., Fujiwara, M., Ozaki, K., Par-khen, L., Mori, T., Primary pineal endodermal sinus tumor with elevated serum and CSF alphafetoprotein levels. Case report. J. Neurosurg. 53 (1980), 244–248.
3. Barber, S. G., Smith, J. A., Hughes, R. C., Melatonin as a tumour marker in a patient with pineal tumour. Br. Med. J. II (1978), 328.
4. Cushing, H., Intracranial Tumours. Notes upon a Series of Two Thousand Verified Cases with Surgical-Mortality Percentages Pertaining Thereto. Springfield, Ill.: Ch. C Thomas. 1932.
5. Ho, K.-L., Rassekh, Z. S., Endodermal sinus tumor of the pineal region. Case report and review of literature. Cancer 44 (1979), 1081–1086.
6. Inoue, Y., Takeuchi, T., Tamaki, M., Nin, K., Hakuba, A., Nishimura, S., Sequential CT observations of irradiated intracranial germinomas. AJR 132 (1979), 361–365.
7. Jenkin, R. D. T., Simpson, W. J. K., Keen, C. W., Pineal and suprasellar germinomas. Results of radiation treatment. J. Neurosurg. 48 (1978), 99–107.
8. Johnson, R. T., Yates, P. O., Clinico-pathological aspects of pressure changes at the tentorium. Acta Radiol. (Stockholm) 46 (1956), 242–249.
9. Kawakami, Y., Yamada, O., Tabuchi, K., Ohmoto, T., Nishimoto, A., Primary intracranial choriocarcinoma. J. Neurosurg. 53 (1980), 369–374.
10. Computertomographie intrakranieller Tumoren aus klinischer Sicht (Kazner, E., Wende, S., Grumme, T., Lanksch, W., Stochdorph, O., eds.). Berlin-Heidelberg-New York: Springer. 1981.
11. Kennaway, D. J., McCulloch, G., Matthews, C. D., Seamark, R. F., Plasma melatonin, luteinizing hormone, follicle-stimulating hormone, prolactin, and corticoids in two patients with pinealoma. J. Clin. Endocrinol. Metab. 49 (1979), 144–145.
12. McGeachie, R. E., Gold, L. H. A., Latchaw, R. E., Periventricular spread of tumor demonstrated by computed tomography. Radiology 125 (1977), 407–410.
13. Osborn, A. G., Daines, J. H., Wing, S. D., The evaluation of ependymal and subependymal lesions by cranial computed tomography. Radiology 127 (1978), 397–401.

14. Pecker, J., Scarabin, J.-M., Faivre, J., Simon, J., Adam, Y., Ramée, M. P., Problèmes diagnostiques et thérapeutiques dans les tumeurs de la région pinéale. Rev. Otoneuroophtalmol. *48* (1976), 225–238.

15. Rao, K. C. V. G., Govindan, S., Intracranial choriocarcinoma. Case report. J. Comput. Assist. Tomogr. *3* (1979), 400–404.

16. Sano, K., Diagnosis and treatment of tumours in the pineal region. Acta Neurochir. (Wien) *34* (1976), 153–157.

17. Stachura, I., Mendelow, H., Endodermal sinus tumor originating in the region of the pineal gland. Ultrastructural and immunohistochemical study. Cancer *45* (1980), 2131–2137.

18. Sullivan, H. G., Harbison, J. W., Becker, D. P., Parinaud's syndrome: cerebrovascular disease as a common etiology: analysis of 16 cases. Surg. Neurol. *6* (1976), 301–305.

19. Sung, D. I., Harisiadis, L., Chang, C. H., Midline pineal tumors and surpasellar germinomas: highly curable by irradiation. Radiology *128* (1978), 745–751.

20. Swischuk, L. E., Bryan, R. N., Double midline intracranial atypical teratomas. A recognizable neuroendocrinologic syndrome. AJR *122* (1974), 517–524.

21. Takeuchi, J., Handa, H., Nagata, I., Suprasellar germinoma. J. Neurosurg. *49* (1978), 41–48.

22. Tavcar, D., Robboy, S. J., Chapman, P. H., Endodermal sinus tumor of the pineal region. Cancer *45* (1980), 2646–2651.

23. Wara, W. M., Fellows, C. F., Sheline G. E., Wilson, C. B., Townsend, J. J., Radiation therapy for pineal tumors and suprasellar germinomas. Radiology *124* (1977), 221–223.

24. Wood, J. H., Zimmerman, R. A., Bruce, D. A., Bilaniuk, L. T., Norris, D. G., Schut, L., Assessment and management of pineal-region and related tumors. Surg. Neurol. *16* (1981), 192–210.

25. Yoshiki, T., Itoh, T., Shirai, T., Noro, T., Tomino, Y., Hamajima, I., Takeda, T., Primary intracranial yolk sac tumor. Immunofluorescent demonstration of alpha-fetoprotein synthesis. Cancer *37* (1976), 2343–2348.

26. Zimmerman, R. A., Bilaniuk, L. T., Wood, J. H., Bruce, D. A., Schut, L., Computed tomography of pineal, parapineal, and histologically related tumors. Radiology *137* (1980), 669–677.

Author's address: Dr. E. Schindler, Department of Neurosurgery, University of Vienna Medical School, Währinger Gürtel 18-20, A-1090 Wien, Austria.

Acta Neurochirurgica, Suppl. 35, 60–64 (1985)

Magnetic Resonance Imaging of Midline Pediatric Cerebral Neoplasms

R. A. Zimmerman

Radiology Department, Hospital of the University of Pennsylvania, Philadelphia, PA, U.S.A.

Summary

Over 80 cases of pediatric cerebral disease including 60 brain tumors, have been studied by low field 0.12 Tesla resistive NMR proton imaging. In addition, experience has been gained with proton imaging on a superconducting high field 1.5 Tesla system. Comparison of NMR images at both field strength, and comparison of the images to those obtained with high resolution CT is made. Examples of how NMR images can help to plan patient management is presented.

Keywords: Brain tumors in children; magnetic resonance imaging; computerized tomography.

Introduction

Magnetic resonance imaging (MRI), although a new medical technology, has already established itself as an important diagnostic step in the evaluation of pediatric brain tumors[1]. Our experience in evaluating pediatric patients by low field resistive MRI and by superconducting high field MRI at the Hospital of the University of Pennsylvania and The Children's Hospital of Philadelphia is presented.

Methods and Material

Between November 1982 and November 1984, 120 pediatric patients (birth to age 18) were examined on a 0.12 Tesla prototype resistive magnetic resonance proton imaging device. The system is housed in a 90 decibel (dB) radiofrequency (RF) shielded room. The bore is 20 inches (50.8 cm) with an aperture of 18 inches (45.7 cm) centrally. The head cone contains the RF coils and is 10 inches (25.4 cm) in diameter. The spin warp method (spatial encoding on X and Y axes) is used for MRI. Data collection was by 3 dimensional (3D) multiplanar methods. Data are acquired on a 128 × 128 matrix and then interpolated to 256 × 256 for display. Slices are between 10 and 13 mm thick. Time per slice is function of the technique used, the repetition time (TR), the matrix size, and the number of data averages per pixel value.

All patients examined on the low field resistive system were studied with the partial saturation (PS) technique. This is because of the better signal to noise ratio and image quality achieved with this approach. Spin echo (SE) studies were inadequate with the low field strength of the system used. The repetition time (TR) for the PS technique was 150 msec. For the multiplanar mode it was possible to collect data for up to 16 sections in either the transverse, coronal, or sagittal planes in 10 minutes. The reconstruction time for the 16 sections is around 20 minutes. Thus, all three planes of section can be obtained of the entire head in a period of 30 minutes of scanning time, but image visualization required an additional hour.

From November 1984 through February 1985, 60 pediatric patients were studied on a 1.5 Tesla General Electric Signa magnetic resonance proton imaging system. In general, the studies were done in all three planes utilizing either a PS or SE technique. Partial saturation images were done with a TR between 600 to 800 msec and a time to echo (TE) from 20 to 25 msec. Spin echo images were done with a TR of 1,500 to 2,500 msec with TEs of between 20 and 80 msec. In a typical spin-echo sequence, images were obtained at 2 echo delays, the second of which was a simple multiple of first. For example, with a TR of 2,000 msec, the images might be performed with a TE of 35 and 70 msec at the same time. The acquisition matrix most often was 128 × 256 (256 × 256 optional) corresponding to a spatial resolution of 1 mm × 0.5 mm. Slice thickness was either 3 mm or 5 mm. A multislice study using the PS technique required 3.3 minutes while a spin-echo sequence with a TR of 2,000 msec required 8.5 minutes. Reconstruction time was rapid so that images were available for review immediately after scanning.

Of the sixty pediatric patients studied on the 1.5 Tesla superconducting system, 25 were examined for neoplasms of the central nervous system.

Distribution of the pediatric central nervous system tumors imaged by both the resistive and superconducting system is given in Table 1.

Results and Discussion

In evaluating pediatric cerebral neoplasms the gold standard in medical imaging is the third or fourth generation CT scan. At the minimum, the contrast enhanced (CE) CT scan with a slice thickness of 10 mm

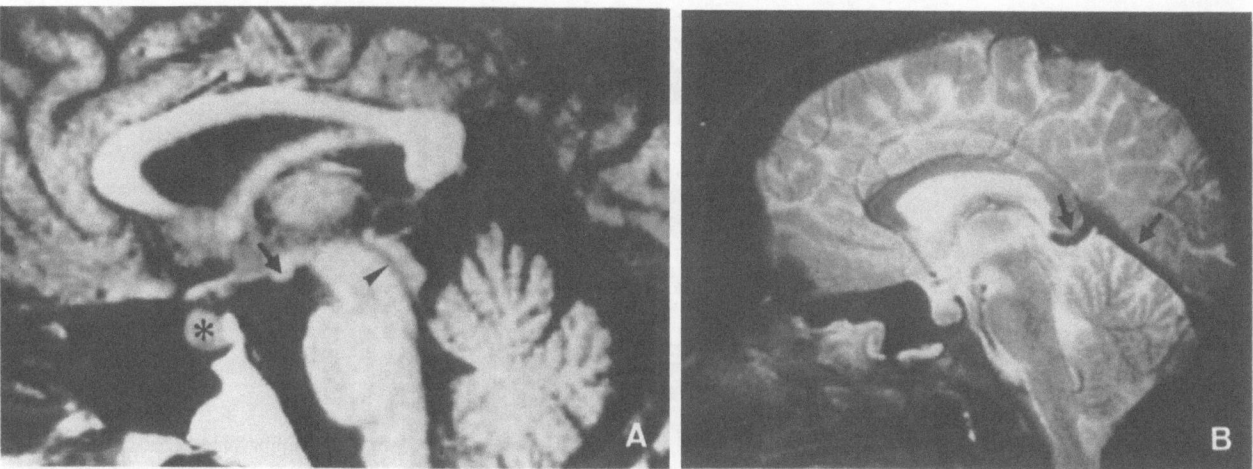

Fig. 1. Normal Anatomy at 1. 5 Tesla. A) 3 mm partial saturation image (TR 800 msec, TE 25 msec). Midline sagittal section (from a series of 9 contiguous slices) shows cerebral aqueduct (arrowhead), mammillary body (arrow), and pituitary gland (asterisk); B) 5 mm spin-echo image (TR 2000 msec, TE 80 msec). Midline sagittal section (from a series of 18 sections, 36 images) shows high signal from CSF, flowing blood in vein of Galen and straight sinus (arrows) produces no signal. Note grey white differentiation within cerebellar folia

or less (5 mm is desirable) is required in pediatrics. It is desirable that a portion of the study be done without enhancement so as to help characterize the tissue (calcification, hemorrhage, hyper-, iso-, hypodensity), and that coronal sections be obtained in specific instances, such as with lesions in and around the sella turcica. The reformating of thin transverse sections into coronal or sagittal images can also prove to be advantageous.

Magnetic resonance imaging has the advantage over CT of involving no ionizing radiation, but in order for MRI to be diagnostically competitive, it must be able to identify lesions with an accuracy similar to that of CT, and the image must also be useful in characterizing and discriminating different types of lesions[6]. The initial experience with MRI relative to CT has been that MRI is much more sensitive than CT. Furthermore, MRI portrays the cerebral neoplasm more graphically in direct images obtained in the coronal, transverse, and sagittal planes. MRI gives clear margins as to the tumor extent and the displacement of the contiguous brain. In posterior fossa tumors, MRI has an inherent edge over CT because of the absence of beam hardening artifacts and artifacts due to axial nonuniformity of the sample volume that frequently degrade the CT image. At present, the specificity of MRI is based primarily upon the location of the tumor, the clinical presentation of the patient, as well as the age and sex. With MRI, calcification is not seen because the protons are nonmobile, a characteristic that is well displayed on CT is lost with MRI. In addition, the phenomena of contrast enhancement as shown with CT are not readily

available with MRI, as paramagnetic contrast agents are not available for clinical use (non-experimental). However, MRI contrast agents such as those using gadolinium will be available in the future.

Fifty-eight out of 80 patients studied on the resistive system and 13 out of 25 patients studied on the superconducting system had midline tumors. In both groups the CT and MRI studies were all positive. The differences were in the qualitative information derived from the various studies. MRI was superior to CT in that it provided high resolution multiplanar imaging of the midline tumor. MRI also had the advantage of greater inherent contrast sensitivity in distinguishing between normal and pathologic brain tissue. The difference in image quality between the high field and low field system related to the relative differences between signal to noise and how that could be applied in producing a higher resolution image with a thinner slice (Figs. 1–5). With the low field system slice thickness was limited to 10 to 13 mm, scanning was limited to the partial saturation technique, and the pixel size was limited to 1 × 1 mm (Fig. 1). With the high field system either the partial saturation or spin-echo technique could be utilized, the slice thickness could be varied from 3 to 10 mm, and the pixel size was 0.5 × 1 mm (Fig. 2). Both the spatial resolution and the contrast sensitivity with the T2 weighted SE image was increased. More importantly, the spin-echo images done with thin sections, of 3 or 5 mm thickness, did not show a degradation in image quality. They both retained morphology and showed the abnormal signal of the pathology. Thus the qualitative information achieved

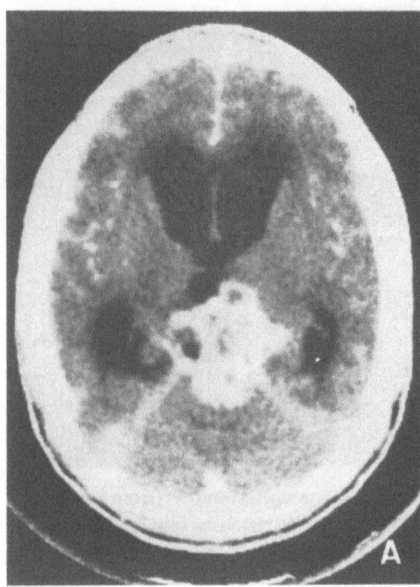 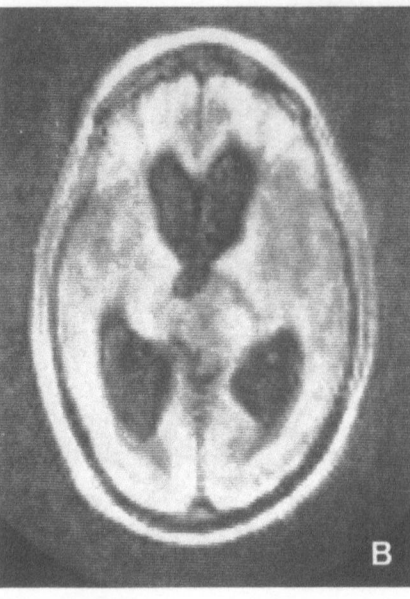

Fig. 2. Embryonal Carcinoma, Pineal Gland. A) Contrast enhanced CT shows pineal mass producing obstructive hydrocephalus; B) MRI study done by partial saturation technique at 0. 12 Tesla shows mass and hydrocephalus

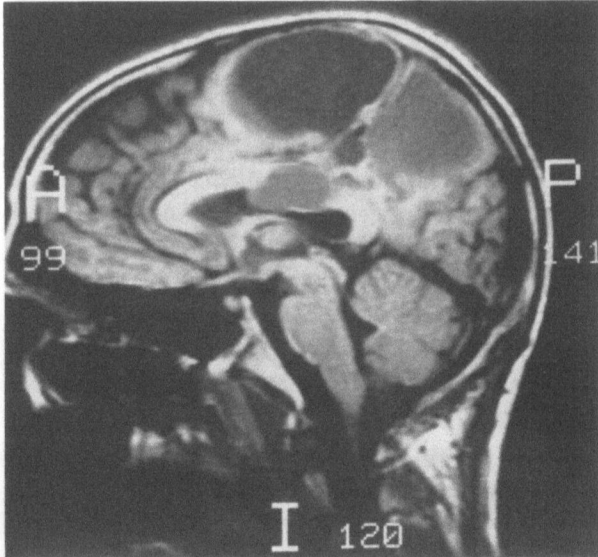

Fig. 3. Cystic Supratentorial Glioma. 5 mm partial saturation image (TR 800 msec, TE 25 msec. 1. 5 Tesla MRI Study. Midline sagittal section shows a necrotic glioma with multiple cysts. Posterior and inferior cysts have higher signal intensities due to higher protein content

at the higher field supplied superior information to that obtained with either the low field MRI system or even to that of the contrast enhanced CT.

It is important to realize that the MRI excelled not only because of lack of artifacts, but also because of the multiple projections used (transverse, coronal, and sagittal planes). Each of these planes of sections contributed to the information provided. In the transverse plane both the lack of artifacts already mentioned

and the increased contrast sensitivity between tissue and CSF are important. In the MRI coronal plane the lack of CT artifacts from filling in teeth, the lack of motion artifacts due to hyperextension of the not fully cooperative head, and the lack of image degradation that accompanies reconstruction of contiguous CT sections made the MRI image more informative. In the direct sagittal MRI image there was exquisitely detailed depiction of the superior, inferior extent of tumor involvement as opposed to the sagittal reconstructed CT image where degradation occurs.

In general, all malignant gliomas of the supratentorial space have been reported to show prolongation of T1 and T2 values relative to normal brain[1,7,8]. Benign tumors have been reported to have T1 and T2 relaxation times shorter than those with malignant tumors[8], but there is overlap so that this finding is not useful in separating the less aggressive tumors from the more malignant tumors[1]. It is believed that the prolongation of relaxation time reflects the relative water content of tissue, relaxation time being proportional to the free water content, and therefore the brighter the image of the tumor (SE), the greater the free water content[9].

Areas of tumor necrosis show prolongation of T1 (Fig. 3) and T2 values. In some instances it may not be possible to separate these areas of necrosis from more solid tumor tissue[8]. Problems also exist in separating edema from tumor tissue. The increased water content of interstitial edema produces prolongation of T1 and T2 values. Contrast between tumor and edema depends on the relative differences in T1 and T2 between the

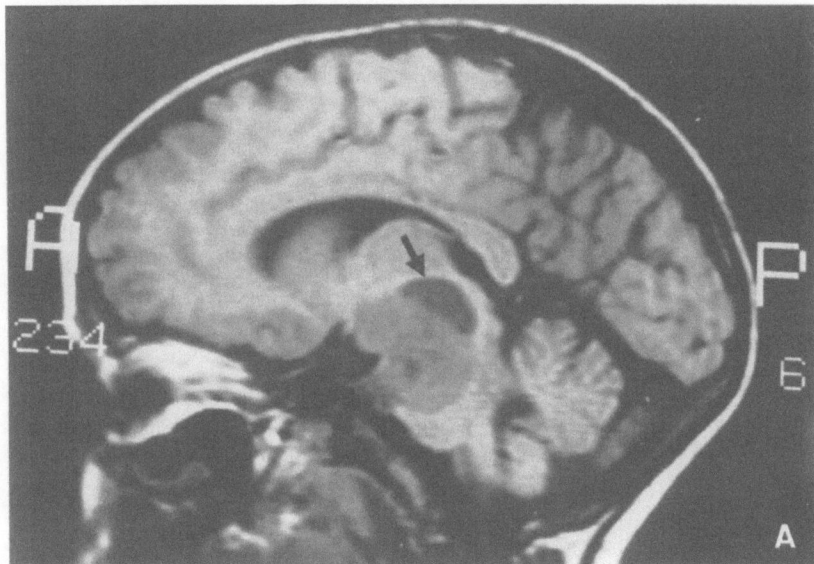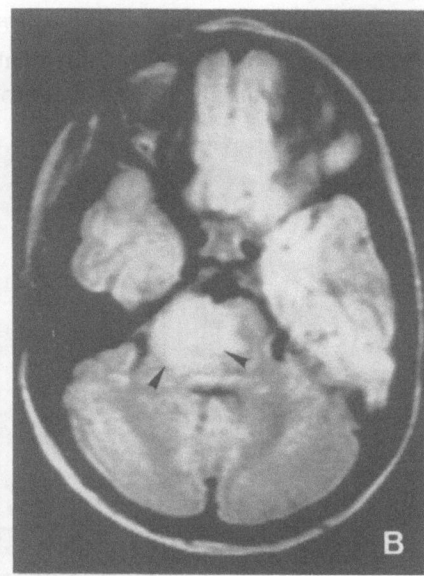

Fig. 4. Brain Stem Glioma. 1. 5 Tesla MRI studies. A) 5 mm partial saturation image (TR 800 msec, TE 25 msec). Sagittal section 5 mm off midline shows a mass (arrowheads) within the upper pons and mesencephalon. Dorsally there is an area of cyst formation (arrow). B) 5 mm spin-echo image (TR 2000 msec, TE 35 msec) high signal mass (arrowheads) in the midpons

tumor and the edema[8]. Thus, it is only where significant differences exist that the tumor and edema will be separable.

Craniopharyngiomas occur in the midline from Rathke's pouch remnants, while epidermoid tumors arise from ectodermal inclusions that cover a wide range of the basilar subarachnoid space and also occur within the calvarium. Ectoderm forms keratin (protein) and cholesterol (fat) debris that is desquamated into the center of the tumor. Relative portions of cholesterol (short T1) and keratin (longer T1) will determine the MRI appearance of the tumor[6]. We have seen a full range of signal intensities with the PS technique in studies of craniopharyngiomas. T1 weighted images are varied in appearance from lesions similar to CSF intensity to those resembling orbital fat. Similar variability was seen in the 5 cases of epidermoid tumors reported in the literature[10,11]. Calcification which occurs in more than 50% of pediatric cranio-pharyngiomas is a characteristic that is lacking in MRI because of the nonmobile nature of the protons in the calcification. Thus, while MRI loses this, MRI does provide other significant advantages in the imaging of craniopharyngiomas. MRI images are direct sections that are not degraded by reconstruction as occurs with CT. The relationship between the craniopharyngioma and important structures such as the optic tracts, hypothalamus, and mesencephalon are well shown with MRI. This information can be critical in the planning of either surgery and/or radiation therapy. This information is important for the radiation therapist in order to design the portal so as to spare the adjacent noninvolved brain tissue.

Approximately 50% of pediatric cerebral neoplasms arise within the posterior fossa. These are either intrinsic to the brain stem or cerebellum, or arise extrinsically within the subarachnoid space or its contiguous structures. Within the brain stem, gliomas are well demonstrated by MRI, with a sensitivity comparable to or better than that of CT (Fig. 4). Zimmerman et al.[4] in evaluating 17 new brain stem gliomas showed MRI to be superior to CT in demonstrating the inferior extent of the tumor into the medulla in 9 of 14 patients (64%) and into the contiguous cervical cord in 5 of 6 patients (83%). Demonstrating the inferior extent of the tumor is important in determining the radiation therapy portals. This can now be done with MRI more accurately and without the invasiveness of intrathecal metrizamide enhanced CT[6]. All authors have reported prolongation of T1 and T2 values in intrinsic gliomas of the brain stem and cerebellum. Packer et al.[3] showed a return to a more normal appearance of the signal intensity at the tumor site following response to radiation therapy. This was at a time when symptoms had remitted and the tumor was reduced in size. Sagittal MRI also proved to be useful in demonstrating enlargement of the brain stem tumor prior to the onset of new symptoms.

Extra-axial tumors are well visualized by MRI. The direction of tumor growth and extent (Fig. 5) prove useful in planning the operative approach.

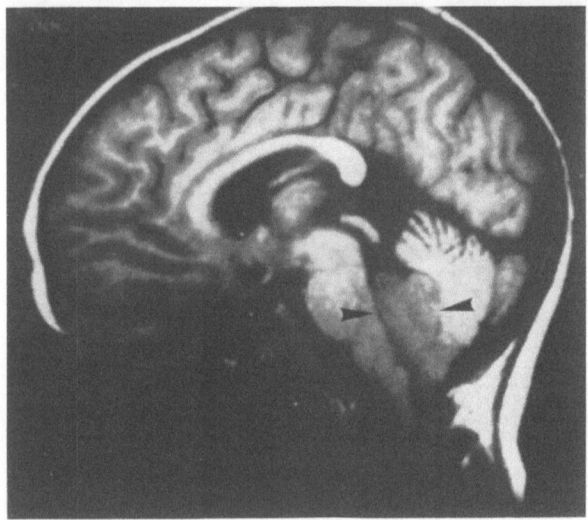

Fig. 5. Ependymoma — 1. 5 Tesla MRI Study. 5 mm midline sagittal partial saturation image shows an intra fourth ventricular mass (arrowheads) growing into the cisterna magna through the foramen of Magendie

Conclusion

MRI, while only available as a diagnostic tool for the past 3 years, has gone through a developmental evolution to become a clinically important tool. This is particularly true for pediatric patients with brain tumors where accurate localization is important in operative planning and in the design and execution of the post- operative radiation therapy.

References

1. Brant-Zawadzki, M., Badami, J. P., Mills, C. M., Norman, D., Newton, T. H., Primary intracranial tumor imaging: a comparison of magnetic resonance and CT. Radiology 150 (1984), 435–440.

2. McGinnis, B. D., Brady, T. J., New, F. J., Buonanno, F. S., Pykett, I. L., De la Paz, R. L., Kistler, J. P., Taveras, J. M., Nuclear magnetic resonance (NMR) imaging of tumors in the posterior fossa. J. Compt. Asst. Tomogr. 7 (1983), 575–584.

3. Packer, R. J., Zimmerman, R. A., Leurson, T. G., Sutton, L. N., Bilaniuk, L. T., Bruce, D. A., Schut, L., Nuclear magnetic resonance in the evaluations of brain stem gliomas of childhood. Neurology (in press).

4. Zimmerman, R. A., Bilaniuk, L. T., Packer, R., Sutton, L., Samuel, L., Johnson, M. H., Grossman, R. I., Goldberg, H. I., Resistive NMR of brain stem gliomas. Neuroradiol. 27 (1985), 21–25.

5. Peterman, S. B., Steiner, R. E., Bydder, G. M., Magnetic resonance imaging of intracranial tumors in children and adolescents. AJNR 5 (1984), 703–709.

6. Zimmerman, R. A., Magnetic resonance imaging of cerebral neoplasms. Magnetic Resonance Annual, pp. 113–144. 1985.

7. Mills C. M., Crooks, L. E., Kaufman, L., Brant-Zawadzki, M., Cerebral abnormalities: use of calculated T1 and T2 magnetic resonance images for diagnosis. Radiology 150 (1984), 87–94.

8. Randell, C. P., Collins, A. G., Young, I. R., Haywood, R., Thomas, D. J., McDonnell, M. J., Orr, J. S., Bydder, G. M., Steiner, R. E., Nuclear magnetic resonance imaging of the posterior fossa tumors. AJNR 4 (1983), 1027–1034.

9. Tsutomu A., Tamon I., Hirokazu, S., Tohru M., Masahiro T., Magnetic resonance imaging of brain tumors: measurement of T1. Radiology 150 (1984), 95–98.

10. Hans, J. S., Bonstelle, C. T., Kaufman, B., Benson, J. E., Alfidi, R. J., Clampitt, M., VanDyke, C., Huss, R. G., Radiology 150 (1984), 705–712.

11. Johnson, M. A., Pennock, J. M., Bydder, G. M., Steiner, R. E., Thomas, D. J., Hayward, R., Bryant, D. R. T., Payne, J. A., Levene, M. I., Whitelaw, A., Dubowitz, L. M. S., Dubowitz, V., Clinical NMR imaging of the brain in children: normal and neurologic disease. AJNR 4 (1983), 1013–1026.

Author's address: Prof. Dr. R. A. Zimmerman, Section Chief, Neuroradiology Section, Hospital of the University of Pennsylvania, 3400 Spruce Street/G 1, Philadelphia, PA 19104, U.S.A.

Acta Neurochirurgica, Suppl. 35, 65–69 (1985)

Neuroimaging of Mass Lesions of the Pineal Region in Infancy and Childhood

P. **Vorkapic** and **G. Pendl**

Department of Neurosurgery, University of Vienna Medical School, Wien, Austria

Summary

Mass lesions of the pineal gland, quadrigeminal plate, posterior third ventricle and midbrain are grouped together as pineal region lesions. The various methods of neuroimaging should not only help to localise and circumscribe these lesions, but should also suggest their quality and nature, i.e. cystic parts, delineation and possible histology. Also, the pathomorphological pattern with respect to the position of the aqueduct and the direction of growth towards the third ventricle and trigone of the lateral ventricle plays an important role in deciding which approach is possible and most suitable. Of major importance are the deep vascular structures and the vasculature of the lesion itself. The study is based on 24 cases of the pediatric age group from a total of 52 observed cases.

Keywords: Pineal region; angiography; ventriculography; CT; NMR.

Introduction

Microneurosurgery of any lesion of the pineal region, in which the posterior third ventricle and midbrain are included, demands a precise preoperative diagnosis including the exact localisation and delineation as well as the vascularity of the lesion and its growth pattern towards the normal vascular structures. CT scanning has much enhanced the early detection of pineal region lesions and has therefore greatly improved the surgical approach. But for planning surgery angiograms still have their merits besides helpfulness in verifying vascular processes like AV malformations. In many cases ventriculography with positive contrast medium will be of importance for evaluating the position and patency of the aqueduct and posterior third ventricle. Nuclear magnetic resonance will become important in the future, although it is not yet available in all centers.

Material and Methods

In the past 12 years, pineal lesions were diagnosed in 24 infants and children aged 3 months to 16 years by various neuroimaging methods. The overall male—female ratio was 15/9. The histology of 20 cases is summarized in Table 1. 4 cases were not subjected to surgery, therefore histology is not known. Table 2 lists the various neuroimaging methods applied. 4 cases were diagnosed in the pre-CT era. Methods are compared in terms of their importance for surgical intervention and later pathomorphological findings.

Table 1. *Histological Distribution of 20 Verified Processes of the Pineal- and Midbrain Region in Children*

	Pineal	Midbrain
Pineocytoma	2	
Germinoma	2	
Pilocytic astrocytoma	1	3
Ependymoblastoma		1
Medulloblastoma		3
Astrocytoma grade II		1
Glial cyst	3	
Glioma (biopsy)		1
PNET	1	
Hamartoma		1
Hematoma		1

Table 2. *Methods of Neuroimaging in 24 Cases of Pineal- and Midbrain-Region Processes in Children.*

	No.	Positive	??	Negative
Native skull X-ray	24	1	2	
Angiography	15	8	1	6
Ventriculography	10	10		
CT	19	17	2	
NMR	1	1		

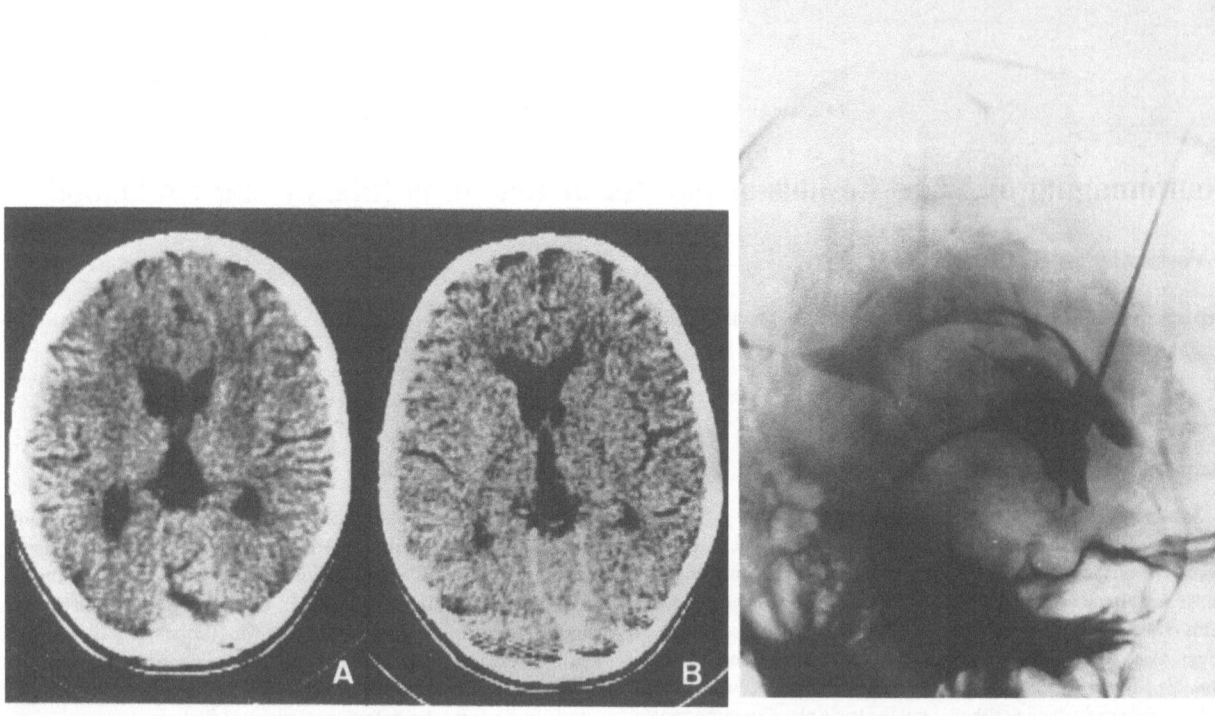

Fig. 1. 12-year-old girl. Pineocytoma of the pineal region. A) CT Scan: A hypodense circumscribed lesion is located in the posterior part of the third ventricle and the pineal region, thus disturbing CSF flow with resultant hydrocephalic enlargement of the lateral ventricles; B) no enhancement of the lesion after application of contrast medium; C) ventriculography with water-soluble contrast medium clearly shows a polycyclically configurated space-occupying lesion originating from the pineal region and bulging into the posterior third ventricle. The aqueduct of Sylvius is in its normal position and patent

Results

CT scanning is the most valuable diagnostic tool for the exact localisation of lesions in the pineal and midbrain regions. The relation of the lesions to the third ventricle, to the splenium of the corpus callosum, the midbrain and the cerebellum is clearly defined in most cases and the most appropriate route for the surgical approach can be chosen. Also, the pathomorphological structure of the lesion was clearly established in all age groups, with information provided on the exact delineation versus normal structures or the infiltrative nature of more malign lesions, although enhancement with contrast media was not always possible. Information on the patency of the aqueduct was only obtainable with additional ventriculography with water-soluble contrast media in cases with hydrocephalic enlargement of the supratentorial ventricular system (Figs. 1 A, B, C). No doubt, NMR will be of great help in such cases (Figs. 2 A, B), but is not widely available yet. A definite diagnosis, including the histological nature, will be possible in cases with glious cysts of the pineal

region. Since the position of the aqueduct relative to the lesion can only be defined by ventriculography in most cases, the involvement of the posterior third ventricle by the mass lesion can equally be seen by this method (Figs. 3, 4). Also, application of water-soluble contrast medium by lumbar puncture in nonhydrocephalic cases shows the cisterns around the midbrain on CT in the presence of rather small lesions.

While angiography reveals vascular malformations in some cases, it is less well suited for differentiating lesions. It provides important information on the vascular supply of the lesion and shows abnormal blood vessels, but visualization of the normal arteries and veins relative to the lesion and their displacement is more important (Fig. 5). In our own series the arterial phase of the angiogram was of minor relevance, except in cases with vascular malformations, such as AV-malformations and vein of Galen aneurysm (Figs. 6 A, 8). By contrast the venous phase of the angiogram was very useful for determining the position of the cortical veins in planning the appropriate surgical approach.

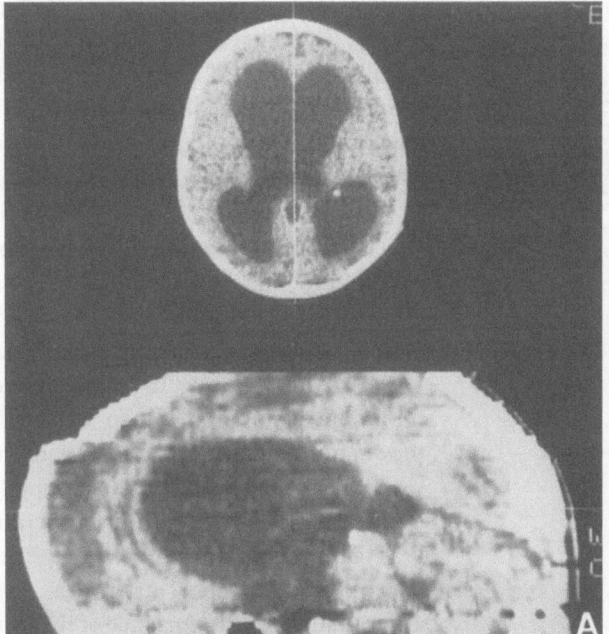
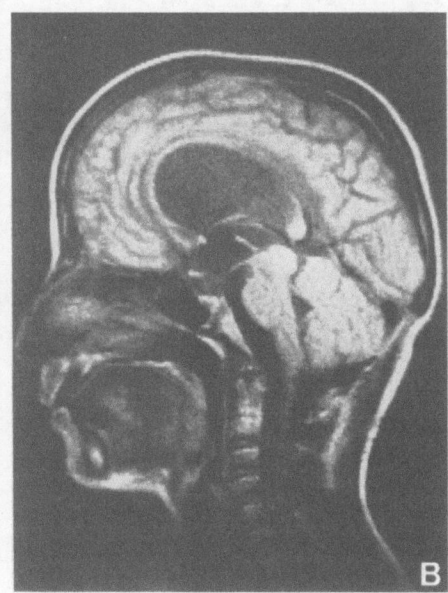

Fig. 2. 13-year-old boy. Glioma of the pineo-mesencephaliç region. A) CAT Scan: Distended dorsal mesencephalon, marked hydrocephalus of the third and the lateral ventricles. No precise information on the nature and localization of the lesion; B) nuclear magnetic resonance image: Distinct well-delineated space-occupying lesion in the dorsal midbrain compressing the aqueduct

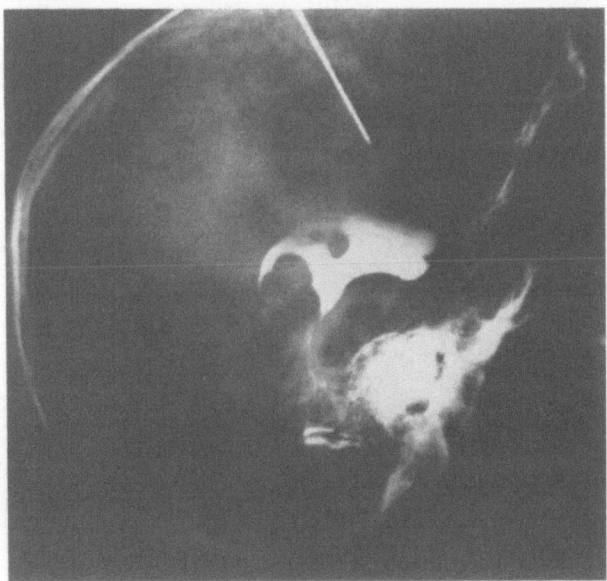

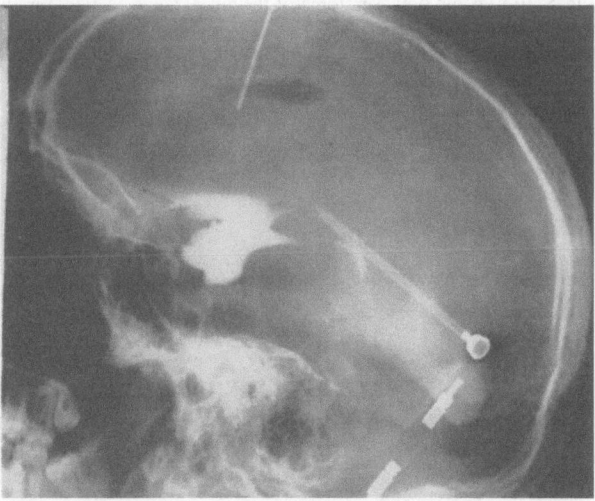

Fig. 4. 16-year-old boy. Pilocytic astrocytoma of the midbrain. Ventriculography with water-soluble contrast medium: There is a filling defect in the posterior third ventricle, the aqueduct is displaced upwards and occluded

Fig. 3. 12-year-old boy. Anaplastic germinomas of the pineal region. Ventriculography with water-soluble contrast medium: Lobulated space-occupying lesion protruding into the posterior third ventricle. The aqueduct is displaced downwards and compressed, but patent

Displacement of deep venous structures, mainly the vein of Galen, internal cerebral veins and basal vein of Rosenthal, shows the growth direction of the lesion and the relationship of these vessels to the lesion (Figs. 7 and 8).

Discussion

Microneurosurgery of lesions in the pineal and midbrain regions demand exact preoperative localization[9, 13, 15]. Most important among neuroimaging technique in these lesion is the CT scan[10]. CT scanning delineate the lesion well enough from the normal structures and also shows the size and growth pattern.

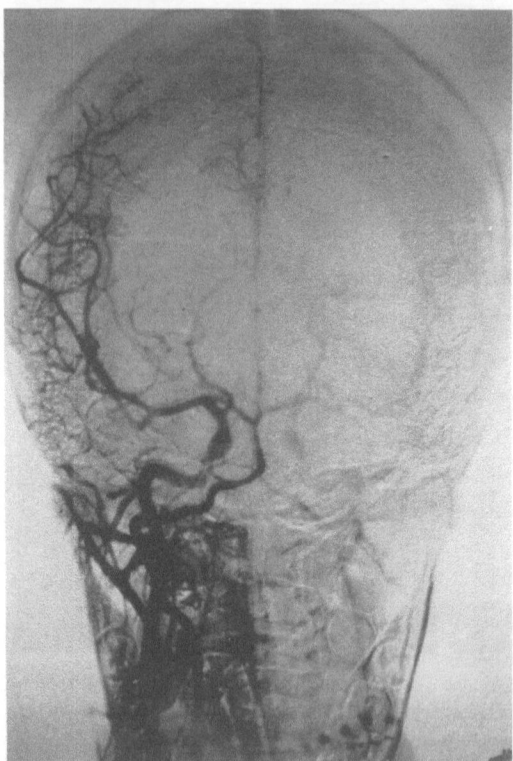

Fig. 5. 10-year-old boy. Teratoma of the pineal gland. Angiography shows arch-shaped distension of the mesencephalic segment of the right posterior cerebral artery

ventricular system and its nature, with possible periventricular hypodensity in pressure hydrocephalus, can equally be seen. CT scans in combination with water-soluble contrast media may show the basal cisterns in axial and extraaxial lesions of the basal midbrain[11] as well as lesions involving the ambient and quadrigeminal cisterns.

To assess the abnormal location of vessels in and around the pineal and midbrain regions, their normal course has to be studied[3, 12, 17]. Angiography and digital subtraction angiograms also show the smaller caliber vessels in this region[6, 7]. In mass lesions of the pineal and midbrain regions the course and position of the posterior choroidal arteries are of major importance along with those of the posterior thalamoperforating arteries. These arteries either feed the lesion or are displaced by it[3, 8]. The veins rather than the arteries determine the appropriate surgical approach. Therefore, most authors stress the importance of the course and position of the deep venous system, i.e. the tributaries to the vein of Galen with the internal cerebral veins and the basal veins of Rosenthal[1, 14]. The position and course of the cortical veins and the dural sinus are equally important for planning the surgical approach. Vascular malformations are the domaine proper at angiography. In

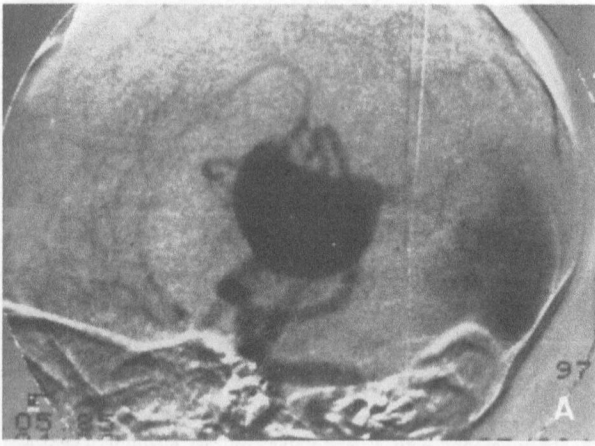 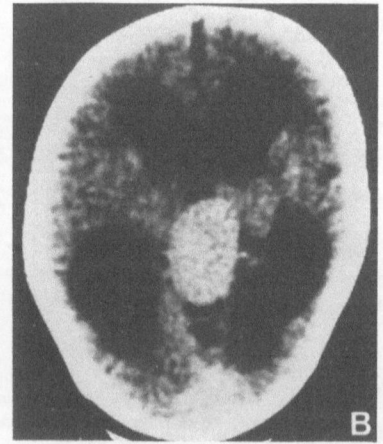

Fig. 6. 3-month-old child. A) intravenous digital subtraction angiography: Great vein of Galen aneurysm. The main arterial feeders originate from the posterior choroidal arteries on both sides; B) CAT scan: Egg-shaped enhancing mass in the pineal region well delineated with markedly hydrocephalic ventricles

In some cases enhancement may tentatively suggest the histological diagnosis preopeatively[16]. Coronal and sagittal reconstructions help determine the relation to the midbrain and third ventricle and the position within the tentorial notch[4]. Identification of the supratentorial extension of the mass is essential for planning the surgical approach. Hydrocephalic enlargement of the

these it is superior to CT scans; in fact it is the only method which provides detailed angiological information of the various pathological patterns so that a rational surgical strategy can be designed[5]. Some authors doubt the need of ventriculography since CT scanning has become available. Not only is it invasive, but it does not offer any further information[18].

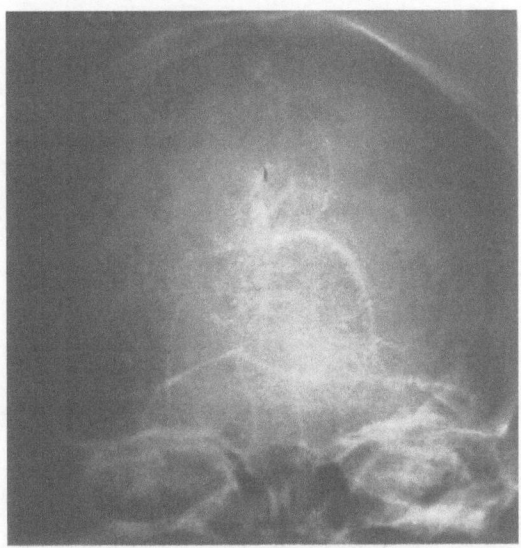

Fig. 7. 14-year-old boy. Glioma of the midbrain. Angiography (a–p view): The basal vein of Rosenthal is displaced laterally and upwards

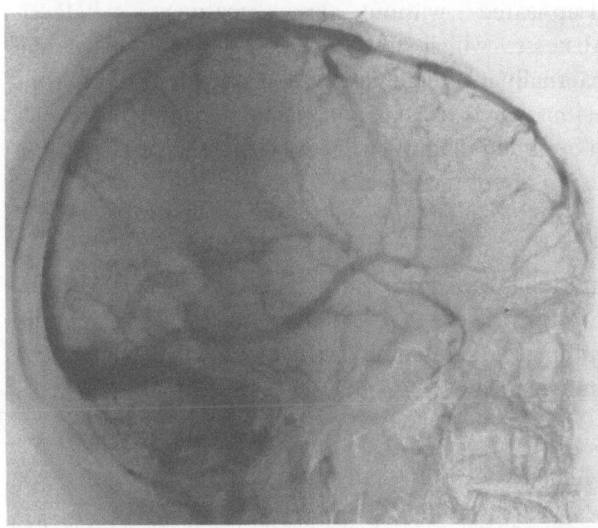

Fig. 8. 16-year-old girl. Pineocytoma of the pineal region. Angiography-venous phase: The vein of Galen is elevated, the basal vein of Rosenthal is displaced anteriorly where it enters the vein of Galen

However, non-enhancing isodense masses are not sufficiently well defined by CT in terms of their relationship to the posterior third ventricle. In small lesions of less than 1.5 cm in diameter intrinsic to the midbrain the position of the aqueduct is of interest, but cannot be seen on CT. Hydrocephalic enlargement of the supratentorial ventricular system can, in some cases, be evaluated by ventriculography, when CT fails to provide useful information on the pineal-midbrain region[2, 7]. NMR will probably replace ventriculography in the future.

References

1. Abay, E. O., Laws, E. R., Grado, G. L., *et al.*, Pineal tumors in children and adolescents. J. Neurosurg. *55* (1981), 889–895.
2. Altenburg, H., Brandt, M., König, H.-J., Ventriculography as a diagnostic procedure in CNS tumors in childhood: its indications and interpretation. In: Tumors of the Central Nervous System in Infancy and Childhood (Voth, D., *et al.*, eds.), pp. 145–148. Berlin-Heidelberg-New York: Springer. 1982.
3. Baker, H. L., The venous angiogram: A frequently overlooked phase of carotid angiography. Clin. Neurosurg. *10* (1964), 297–310.
4. Delavelle, J., Megret, M., CT sagittal reconstruction of posterior fossa tumors. Neuroradiology *19* (1980), 81–88.
5. Diebler, C., Dulac, O., Renier, D., Ernest, C., Lalande, G., Aneurysms of the vein of Galen in infants aged 2 to 15 months. Diagnosis and natural evolution. Neuroradiology *21* (1981), 185–195.
6. Duvernoy, H. M., Human Brain Stem Vessels. Berlin-Heidelberg-New York: Springer. 1978.
7. Fitz, C. R., Harwood-Nash, D. C., Chuang, S., Resjo, M. I., Metrizamid ventriculography and computed tomography in infants and children. Neuroradiology *16* (1978), 6–9.
8. Hase, U., Hock, H., Schindler, E., Tumoren der Pinealisregion. Neurochirurgie *22* (1979), 107–117.
9. Ismat, F., Tumors of the posterior part of the third ventricle: neurosurgical criteria. In: Advances and Technical Standards in Neurosurgery, Vol. 6 (Krayenbühl, H., *et al.*, eds.), pp. 171–184. Berlin-Heidelberg-New York: Springer. 1979.
10. Kazner, E., Wende, S., Grumme, Th., Lanksch, W., Stochdorph, O., Computertomographie intrakranieller Tumoren, pp. 189–197. Berlin-Heidelberg-New York: Springer. 1981.
11. McAllister, V. L., Hankinson, J., Sengupta, R. P., Problems in diagnosis with computerized tomography. In: Advances in Neurosurgery, Vol. 6 (Wüllenweber, R., *et al.*, eds.), Berlin-Heidelberg-New York: Springer. 1978.
12. Pachtman, H., Hilal, S. K., Wood, E. H., The posterior choroidal arteries. Normal measurements and displacement by hydrocephalus and tumors of the pineal region or brain stem. Radiology *112* (1974), 343–352.
13. Pendl, G., Mikrotopographische Untersuchungen über die operativen Zugänge zur Mittelhirn-Pinealisregion. Habilitationsschrift, Wien, 1980.
14. Reid, W. S., Clark, K. W., Comparison of the infratentorial and transtentorial approaches to the pineal region. Neurosurgery *3* (1978), 1–8.
15. Stein, B. M., Surgical Treatment of Pineal Tumors. (Clin. Neurosurg., Vol. 269), pp. 491–510. Baltimore: Williams & Wilkins. 1979.
16. Ueki, K., Tanaka, R., Treatment and prognosis of pineal tumors. Experience of 110 cases. Neurol. Med. Chir. (Tokyo) *20* (1980), 1–26.
17. Wackenheim, A., Braun, P., Angiography of the Mesencephalon. Berlin-Heidelberg-New York: Springer. 1970.
18. Wende, S., Do we need ventriculography in the era of computed tomography? Neuroradiology *23* (1982), 89–90.

Author's address: Dr. P. Vorkapic, Department of Neurosurgery, University of Vienna Medical School, Währinger Gürtel 18-20, A-1090 Wien, Austria.

Acta Neurochirurgica, Suppl. 35, 70–74 (1985)

CT Stereotactic Biopsy for Optimizing the Therapy of Intracranial Processes

F. Mundinger

Department of Stereotaxy and Neuronuclear Medicine, Neurochirurgische Universitätsklinik Freiburg, Federal Republic of Germany

Summary

The CT stereotactic method (Mundinger/Birg) and the bioptic results of intracranial processes in 815 cases are reported. In 17% of the cases, no tumor was found, in contrast to the diagnosis established by modern imaging techniques (CT, MRI). The necessity of confirming the diagnosis of intracranial lesions to optimize the treatment plan is pointed out. Low mortality and morbidity rates (0.6 and 3%) make this method acceptable for the patient, since misdiagnoses, mistreatment or omission of treatment can thus be avoided. The accuracy (0.6 mm) of CT stereotactic localization and biopsy makes the method reliable even for small lesions.

Keywords: CT stereotactic operation; biopsy; Curietherapy.

Introduction

With modern image-producing techniques such as X-Ray Transmission Computer Tomography (CT) and Magnetic Resonance Imaging (MRI) it is possible to accurately and reliably locate intracranial processes. But with regard to a morphological diagnosis, the initial enthusiasm for these procedures has been replaced by a certain disillusionment. We have been able to show, in fact, that 164 out of 904 intracranial lesions which we stereotactically biopsied and which had been previously diagnosed as tumors because of their ring structures, were bioptically found to be no tumors at all[18, 23, 24]. In addition, multiple foci which had been diagnosed as metastases on the CT scan[25, 33]—as well as by MRI—were bioptically found to be multiple hemorrhages, abscesses or even multiple sclerotic lesions, but no metastases.

Processes which are surgically non-resectable, located at the base of the skull or in the midline area and presumed to be tumors are still treated conservatively or by external radiation without a prior histological diagnosis. In the literature the treatment of processes in the diencephalon, mesencephalon and brainstem/pons region is either described as unsuccessful or excellent results are reported for radiotherapy of "tumors" which were actually cysts, necroses, glioses, etc. and would have remained unchanged or would even have disappeared without any treatment whatever. Abscesses which are found by the pathologist and externally irradiated as "tumors" or multiple sclerotic lesions which, because of this treatment and the absence of optimum therapy, will deteriorate or actually lead to death, are critical cases.

CT stereotactic biopsy[1, 2, 3, 6, 7, 8, 9, 10, 11, 16, 26, 27, 28, 30, 31, 32, 34], however, succeeds in establishing an accurate and reliable histological diagnosis. Together with the intraoperative diagnosis by smears this helps to optimize therapeutic measures and take them immediately.

Method

For carrying out CT stereotactic biopsy we use our own stereotactic device (Riechert/Mundinger[29]) in a computer-compatible version (Mundinger/Birg[20, 23]). Its principles and technique have been described elsewhere[4, 5, 18, 24]. Through the same burrhole of 7 mm in diameter, several puncture tracks have to be made in different directions, using the transcerebral or transcerebellar approaches (Fig. 1). The accuracy of location is 0.6 mm[23, 24].

Our biopsies are carried out with biopsy forceps of 0.8 mm in diameter, which are guided in a 1.0 mm diameter cannula. Step by step, in intervals of millimeters, tissue of about $1/3$ mm^3 volume is taken. This amount of tissue is sufficient for histological purposes[12, 13, 18]. Material is taken from the same site for both intraoperative histology by smears and conventional examination. The biopsy needle is directed from the perifocal area through the lesion so that the marginal areas are included. If only amorphous material is found, the differentiation between non-tumor associated necroses, e.g. those caused by hemorrhage or infarction, and those caused by the tumor is especially difficult. In these cases, the marginal area is tangentially examined by additional bioptic tracks. By using this method, a morphological profile of the lesion is established. This is most important for establishing the malignancy of the tumor.

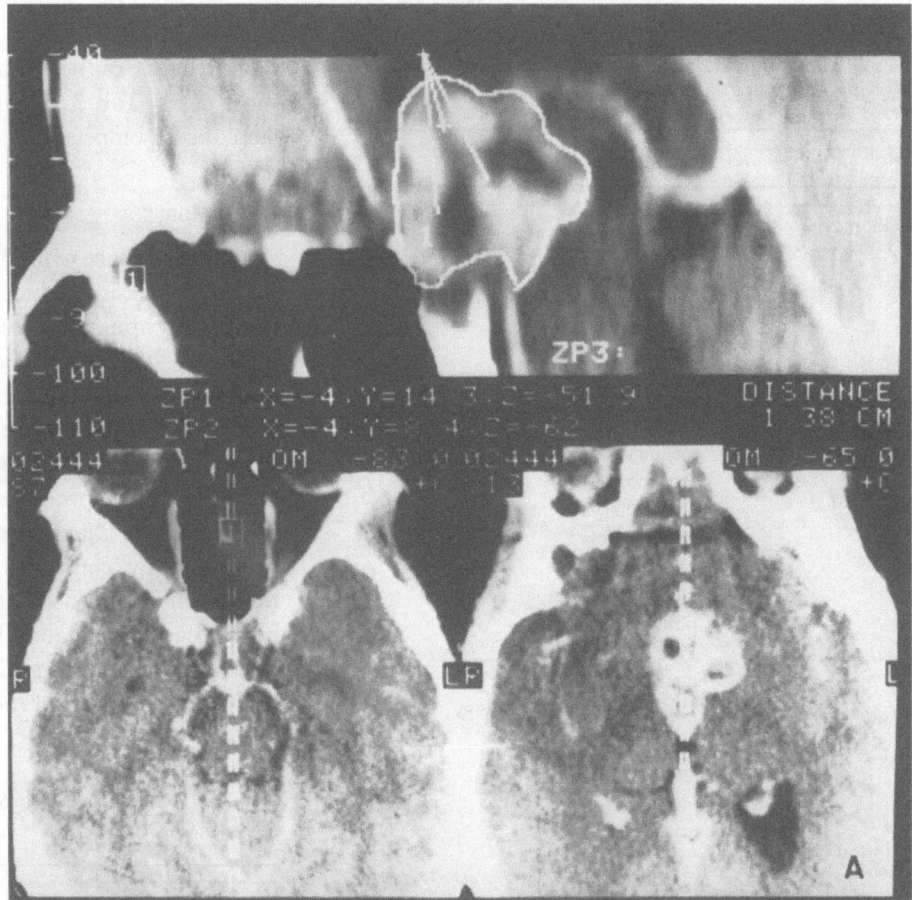

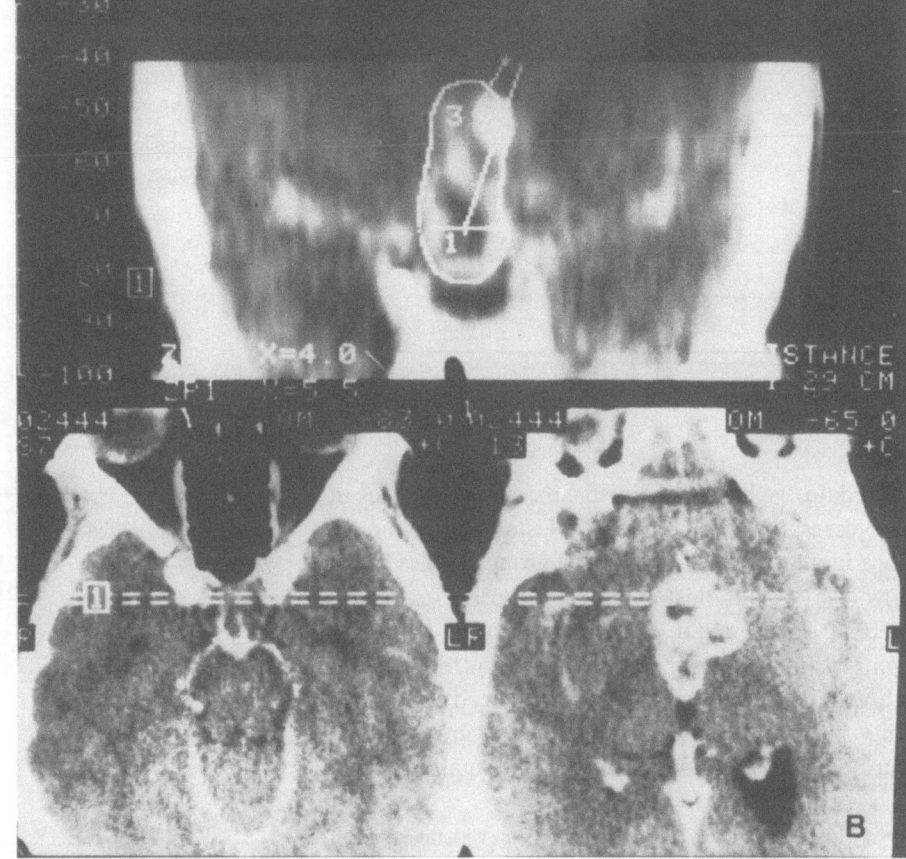

Fig. 1. Gemistocytic astrocytoma, WHO Grade II. After attaching the stereotactic base ring to the patient's head and making the coordinate axes "stereotactic ring/CT gantry" coincide, parallel scans are taken with enhancement. The zero section is situated in the centre of the base ring so that all the coordinate measures in CT are, at the same time, those to the stereotactic system. A) sagittal reconstruction through astrocytoma showing predominantly hyperdense demarcation and calcifications, and puncture tracks for biopsy and subsequent implantation of Iodine-125 seeds (ZY coordinates); B) coronal reconstruction showing tumor extension, planned biopsy tracks and implantation sites (X coordinates)

Table 1. *Intraoperative Diagnosis of CT-Stereotactic Biopsy in the Smear Preparation (January 1981–June 30, 1984)*

Histological diagnosis		Cases
a) Gliomas	astrocytoma I	81
	astrocytoma II	213
	astrocytoma III	123
	glioblastoma IV	64
	oligodendroglioma	25
		515
b) Non glial tumors	meningioma	9
	germinoma	17
	craniopharyngioma	27
	ependymoma	7
	plexuspapilloma	4
	medulloblastoma	5
	pituitary adenoma	10
	PNET	21
	metastasis	55
	tumor of unknown etiology	6
	colloid—cyst	6
		167
c) No tumors	necrosis	9
	gliosis	42
	abscess	12
	angioma	2
	hemorrhage	28
	infarction	10
	inflammation of ventricle	1
	encephalitis	2
	stenosis of aqueductus sylvii	3
	mucocele	1
	arachnoid cyst	20
	no tumor	3
		133
	total	815

Results

To date, we have performed stereotactic biopsies in 1,293 cases, including 815 with CT stereotactic biopsy (since January 1981)*. For the last group, Tables 1a–1c show the bioptic histological diagnoses for intracerebral, extracerebral, intracranial tumors and non-tumor lesions which appeared to be tumors on imaging. Tab. 2 indicates mortality and morbidity rates. Morbidity is usually characterized by an aggravation of neurological symptoms. It is caused by small localized

---

* I wish to thank Dr. K. Weigel for helping me with the statistics.

hemorrhages or perifocal edema and is transient in most cases. Tab. 3 shows the therapies following CT stereotactic biopsies.

Discussion

Our experience with CT stereotactic biopsies showed that 17% of lesions which were previously diagnosed as tumors by imaging techniques are, in fact, non-tumorous. Our results suggest that, considering the minimal risk and high reliability of the bioptic procedure, no conservative or percutaneous radiation therapy should be carried out today in patients with space-occupying processes without a previous histological diagnosis. Diagnostic errors, especially the wrong or no therapy, can thus be avoided. In non-resectable tumors or recurrences and/or external radiation, the biopsy can immediately be followed by local therapy within the same sitting. Depending on the malignancy of the tumor, different radioactive isotopes are perma-

Table 2. *Complications After Stereotactic Biopsy (1,293 Cases)—1965–June 30, 1984*

	No. of cases	(%)
Operative mortality	8	0.6
Operative morbidity		
transient complications	52	4
persistent complications	33	3
Type of complications		
hemorrhage	26	2
paresis	25	2
aphasia	16	1
seizure	38	3

Table 3. *Type of Subsequent Treatment After Stereotactic Diagnostic Biopsy (1965–June 30, 1984)*

Type of procedure		No. of cases	(%)
Permanent interstitial			
Curietherapy	Ir-192	254	20
	J-125	298	23
+ External irradiation		78	7
Temporary interstitial			
(brachy-)Curietherapy		75	7
External irradiation		215	17
Cyst drainage			
(catheter implantation)		88	7
Tumor resection		79	6
No subsequent therapy		389	30

nently implanted (Curie therapy). In low-grade tumors we have used Iridium-192 since 1959 and Iodine-125 since 1979. For high-grade tumors, temporary interstitial or intracavitary radiation in terms of afterloading with the Iridium-192 contact radiation device "GammaMed" (R) has been used since 1963 or, alternatively, Iodine-125 catheter systems[17, 18, 19, 21, 22, 25, 33] since 1979. Drainage of cysts, irrigation of abscesses and ventricular shunts are further stereotactic indications which can be carried out during the same operation. Therefore this method offers optimum management, as documented by our results.

The nature of the tumor is of decisive importance especially in cases where external radiation therapy and possibly treatment with cytostatic agents are considered. Patients suffering from anaplastic gliomas (WHO III) have a longer life-expectancy than those with glioblastomas (WHO IV). Low-grade tumors (WHO I, II) are, to a great extent, resistant to external radiation up to 65 Gy[14, 15]. In addition, histological confirmation is absolutely indispensable for statistical evaluation of tumor treatment methods, particularly in midline, diencephalic, mesencephalic, quadrigeminal plate and brainstem/pons tumors.

While the instrument for biopsy should be as small as possible, they should provide for the removal of adequately large tissue fragments to ensure diagnostic accuracy. The difference in mortality and complication rates can be accounted for by the differences in the instruments used[2, 8, 16, 30, 31].

The low complication rates for operations carried out with our CT-assisted stereotactic technique (mortality 0.6%, morbidity: transient 4%, persistent 3%) make this method acceptable for the patient.

References

1. Apuzzo, M. L. J., Zelman, V., Jepson, J., Chandrasoma: Observations with the utilization of the Brown-Roberts-Wells stereotactic system in the management of intracranial mass lesions. Acta Neurochir. Suppl. *33* (1984), 261–263.

2. Backlund, E. O., A new instrument for stereotaxic brain tumour biopsy. Acta Chir. Scand. *137* (1971), 825–827.

3. Bergstroem, M., Greitz, T., Steiner, I., An approach to stereotactic radiography. Acta Neurochir. *54* (1980), 157–165.

4. Birg, W., Mundinger, F., Computer calculations of target parameters for a stereotactic apparatus. Acta Neurochir. *29* (1973), 123–129.

5. Birg, W., Mundinger F., Klar, M., Computer assistance for stereotactic brain operations. Advanc. Neurosurg. *4* (1977), 287–291.

6. Broggi, G., Franzini, A., Giorgi, C., Allegranza, A., Diagnostic accuracy and multimodal approach in stereotactic biopsies of deep brain tumours. Acta Neurochir. Suppl. *33* (1984), 211–212.

7. Brown, R. A., Roberts, T., Osborne, A. T., Simplified CT-guided stereotaxic biopsy. AJNR *2* (1981), 181–184.

8. Daumas-Duport, C., Monsaingeon, V., N'Guyen, J. P., Missir, O., Szikla, G., Some correlations between histological and CT aspects of cerebral gliomas contributing to the choice of significant trajectories for stereotactic biopsies. Acta Neurochir. Suppl. *33* (1984), 185–194.

9. Galanda, M., Nadvornik, P., Sramka, M., Basandova, M., Stereotactic biopsy of brainstem tumors. Acta Neurochir. Suppl. *33* (1984), 213–217.

10. Kelly, P. J., Kall, B. A., Goerss, S.G., *et al.*, Stereotactic surgery for CNS tumours & G. E. notes. CT Clinical Symposium Vol. 5 No. *5* (1982).

11. Kelly, P. J., Kall, B. A., Goeras, S. G., Computer assisted stereotactic biopsies utilizing CT and digitized arteriographic data. Acta Neurochir. Suppl. *33* (1984), 233–235.

12. Kiessling, M., Anagnostopoulos, J., Lombeck, G., Kleihues, P., Diagnostic potential of stereotactic biopsy of brain tumours. A report of 400 cases. In: Tumours of the Central Nervous System in Infancy and Childhood (Voth, D., Gutjahr, P., Langmaid, C., eds.), pp. 247–256. Berlin-Heidelberg-New York: Springer. 1982.

13. Kiessling, M., Kleihues, P., Gessaga, E., Mundinger, F., Ostertag, Ch. B., Weigel, K., Morphology and adjacent brain structures following interstitial iodine-125 radiotherapy. Acta Neurochir. Suppl. *33* (1984), 281–289.

14. Kuhlendahl, H., Miltz, H., Wüllenweber, R., Die Astrocytome des Großhirns. Acta Neurochir. *29* (1973), 151–162.

15. Laws, E. R., jr., Taylor, W. F., Marvin, B. C., Okazaki, H., Neurosurgical management of low-grade astrocytoma of the cerebral hemisphere. J. Neurosurg. *651* (1984), 665–673.

16. Monsaingeon, V., Daumas-Duport, C., Mann, M., Miyahara, S., Szikla, G., Stereotactic sampling biopsies in a series of 268 consecutive cases—validity and technical aspects. Acta Neurochir. Suppl. *33* (1984), 195–200.

17. Mundinger, F., The treatment of brain tumors with interstitially applied radioactive isotopes. In: Radionuclide Applications in Neurology and Neurosurgery (Wang, Y., Paoletti, P., eds.), pp. 199–265. Springfield, Ill.: Ch. C Thomas. 1970.

18. Mundinger, F., CT-stereotactic biopsy of brain tumours. In: Tumours of the Central Nervous System in Infancy and Childhood (Voth, D., Gutjahr P., Langmaid, C., eds.), pp. 234–246. Berlin-Heidelberg-New York: Springer. 1982.

19. Mundinger, F., Implantation of radioisotopes (Curie-Therapy). In: Stereotaxy of the Human Brain, 2. Aufl. (Schaltenbrand, C., Walker, A. E., eds.), pp. 410–435. Stuttgart: Thieme. 1982.

20. Mundinger, F., Introduction. P. Dyck: Stereotactic Biopsy and Brachytherapy of Brain Tumors, pp. 9–11. Baltimore: University Park Press. 1984.

21. Mundinger, F., Stereotaktische intrakranielle Bestrahlung von Tumoren mit Radioisotopen (Curie-Therapie). In: Klinische Neurochirurgie. Band II: Klinik und Therapie (Dietz, H., Umbach, W., Wüllenweber, R., eds.), pp. 519–565. Stuttgart-New York: Thieme. 1984.

22. Mundinger, F., Technik und Ergebnisse der interstitiellen Hirntumorbestrahlung. In: Handbuch der medizinischen Radiologie. Band XIX/4: Spezielle Strahlentherapie maligner Tumoren (Heilmann, H. P., ed.), pp. 179–214. Berlin-Heidelberg-New York-Tokyo: Springer. 1985.

23. Mundinger, F., Birg, W., CT-Stereotaxy is the clinical routine. Neurosurg. Rev. *7* (1984), 219–224.

24. Mundinger, F., Birg, W., Stereotactic biopsy of intracranial processes. Acta Neurochir. Suppl. *33* (1984), 219–224.

25. Mundinger, F., Weigel, K., Mohadjer, M., CT-stereotaktische Biopsie und/oder interstitiell-extern kombinierte Strahlenbehandlung von Hirnmetastasen. In: Hirnmetastasen. Pathophysiologie, Diagnostik und Therapie (Aktuelle Onkologie, Vol. 13.) (von Heyden, H. W., Krauseneck, P., eds.), pp. 128–143. München: Zuckschwerdt. 1984.

26. Ohye, C., Nakajima, H., Matsushima, T., Komatsu, T., Hirato, M., Kawashima, Y., CT assisted stereotactic biopsy of deep cerebral lesions and the results. Acta Neurochir. Suppl. *33* (1985), 257–259.

27. Pecker, J., Scarabin, J. M., Brucher, J. M., Vallee, B., Demarche stereotaxique en neurochirurgie tumorale. pp. 1–301. Paris: Pierre Fabre. 1979.

28. Perry, J. H., Rosenbaum, A. E., Lunsford, L. D. *et al.* , Computed tomography-guided stereotactic surgery: conception and development of a new stereotactic methology. Neurosurg. *7* (1980), 376–381.

29. Riechert, T., Mundinger, F., Bechreibung und Anwendung eines Zielgerätes für stereotaktische Hirnoperationen (2. Modell). Acta Neurochir. *3* (1956), 308–337.

30. Scerrati, M., Rossi, G. F., The reliability of stereotactic biopsy. Acta Neurochir. Suppl. *33* (1984), 201–205.

31. Sedan, R., Peragut,J. C., Farnarier, Ph., Hassoun, J., Sethian, M., Intra-encephalic stereotactic biopsies (309 patients/318 biopsies). Acta Neurochir. Suppl. *33* (1984), 207–210.

32. Suetens, P., Gybels, J., Jansen, P., Oosterlinck, A., Haegemans, A., Dierckx, P., A global 3-D image of the blood vessels. Tumor and simulated electrode. Acta Neurochir. Suppl. *33* (1984), 225–232.

33. Weigel, K., Mohadjer, M., Mundinger, F., CT-Stereotaxie zur Differentialdiagnose und interstitiellen Curie-Therapie intrakranieller Metastasen. 34. Jahrestagung der Deutschen Gesellschaft für Neurochirurgie. Mannheim, 27.–30. April 1983.

34. Wise, B. L., Gleason, C., CAT scan-directed stereotactic brain biopsy: With template produced by computer graphics. Acta Neurochir. Suppl. *33* (1984), 265–267.

Author's address: Prof. Dr. F. Mundinger, Medical Director, Department of Stereotaxy and Neuronuclear Medicine, Neurochirurgische Universitätsklinik, Hugstetter Strasse 55, D-7800 Freiburg i. Br., Federal Republic of Germany.

Acta Neurochirurgica, Suppl. 35, 75–79 (1985)
© by Springer-Verlag 1985

F. Lateral and Third Ventricle

Supratentorial Intraventricular Tumors in Childhood

H. Collmann, E. Kazner, and **C. Sprung**

Neurochirurgische Abteilung, Klinikum Charlottenburg, Freie Universität Berlin

Summary

We report on a series of 21 infants and children with tumors of the supratentorial ventricular system, all of whom were assessed by computed tomography and underwent operation using microsurgical techniques. In 7 cases the tumor was found in the 3rd ventricle, whereas the lateral ventricles were involved in the others. Surgical access to the lateral ventricles and the anterior portion of the 3rd ventricle was gained by standard intergyral cortical incision in the precentral or postcentral regions and via the foramen of Monro. The posterior portions of the lateral ventricle of the dominant hemisphere as well as the posterior part of the 3rd ventricle were exposed with minimal risk, using the occipital midsagittal supratentorial route. Following this technique, total removal of the tumors was possible in all cases without substantial postoperative morbidity. After a follow-up period of 6 months to 9 years all patients are in good or excellent neurological condition. Tumor recurrences were not encountered, although a definitive statement cannot be made in some patients with malignant lesions.

Keywords: Ventricular tumors; tumors in tuberous sclerosis.

Introduction

Microsurgical techniques and computerized tomography introduced about ten years ago have both substantially improved the prognosis of intraventricular tumors and lesions. Until then direct surgical attack on these lesions carried a high mortality and morbidity[2, 14, 16, 17, 19], although there are some early reports on successful removal even of tumors within the third ventricle[2, 15]. The profound change in the management of intraventricular tumors gave rise to the present study reviewing the clinical data and CT findings as well as the postoperative outcome in young patients who were operated on during the last decade.

Patients and Methods

The study comprised 21 children and adolescents with tumors and lesions of the supratentorial ventricular system who, except one, were operated on by the second author at the neurosurgical departments of Munich (cases no. 1–9) and Berlin-Charlottenburg after 1975. Prior to operation all of them were submitted to computerized tomography and, during the last year, also to NMR imaging. In each case an attempt was made to predict the histological type of the lesion. Table 1 and Fig. 1 summarize the clinical data of the patients and the CT findings. In 14 cases the lesion was located within the lateral ventricles, the remaining 7 originated within the third ventricle. Histological analysis of surgical specimens revealed 18 benign lesions and tumors and 3 malignant tumors. [The typical age distribution was found in the four cases of plexus papillomas (Tab. 1, Fig. 1 A) and in the patients with subependymal giant cell astrocytoma (Tab. 1, Fig. 1 B).] Since most intraventricular tumors cause high-pressure hydrocephalus the vast majority of our patients presented with signs of raised intracranial pressure. Seizures and focal neurological signs were observed more often in tumors of the lateral ventricles.

Computerized tomography was the diagnostic method of choice in all patients. Most recently magnetic resonance imaging provided additional valuable information on the location and the attachment of the lesion to the ventricular walls. Thus, ventriculography was abandoned and even conventional angiography proved to be unnecessary in nearly all cases. On the basis of clinical data and CT findings a type-specific diagnosis could be established in 16 patients prior to operation. This was particularly true in plexus papillomas, subependymomas and giant cell astrocytomas, most of them originating within the lateral ventricles, while only two out of seven lesions of the third ventricle could be classified preoperatively.

Our series includes seven patients with subependymal giant cell astrocytoma, the characteristic tumor in tuberous sclerosis (Fig.1 B and 2). In all of them the tumors were diagnosed preoperatively, although the classical clinical triad of tuberous sclerosis—adenoma sebaceum, seizures and mental retardation—was found in only two of them and in two others phakomatosis was completely unknown until the CT scan was taken.

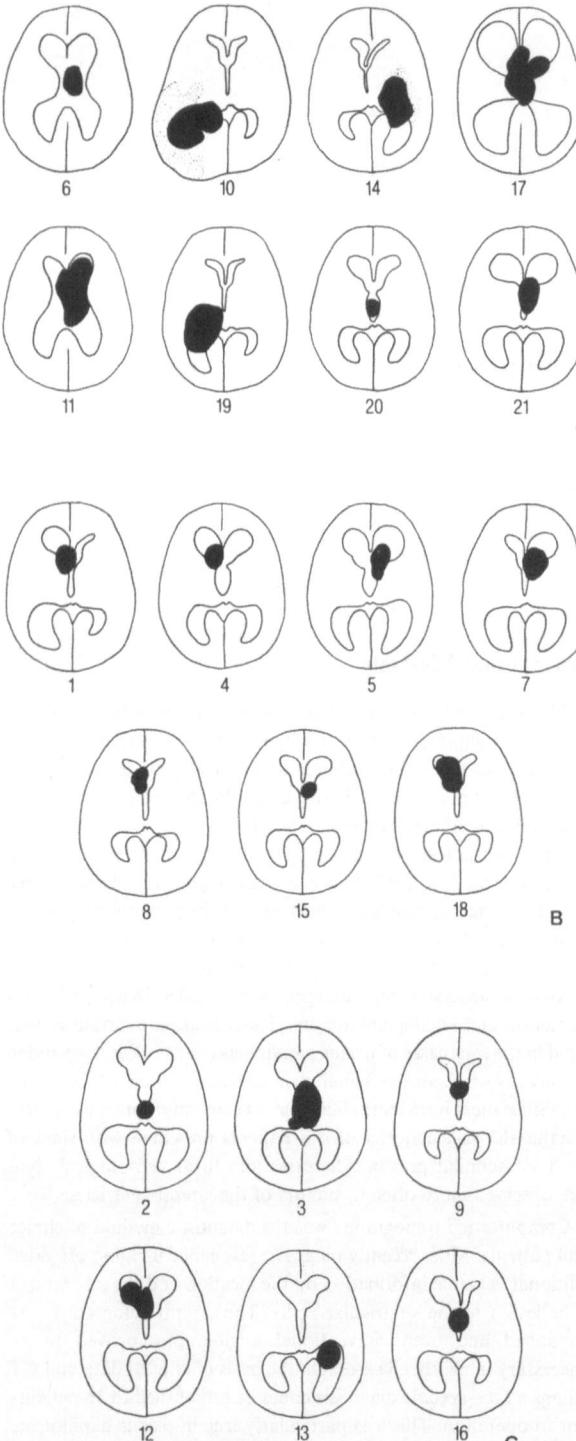

Fig. 1. Schematical reproduction of CT findings in children and adolescents with intraventricular tumors and lesions. Numbers represent cases as indicated in Table 1. Dotted areas = perifocal edema. A) Above: 4 cases of benign (No. 6, 10, 17) and malignant (No. 14) plexus papillomas, below: 2 cases of subependymomas (No. 11, 19), 2 cases of ependymoblastomas (No. 20, 21); B) 7 cases of subependymal giant cell astrocytomas; C) 6 cases of miscellaneous tumors and lesions: Pineocytoma (No. 2), teratoma (No. 3), colloid cyst (No. 9), cavernoma (No. 12), plexus cyst (No. 13), meningioma (No.16).

Surgical Procedures

In this series the frontal and the parietal transcortical approach using the standard intergyral incision was preferred in the majority of patients to enter the lateral ventricles as well as the anterior part of the third ventricle. A precentral transcallosal approach was used in one single case, but resulted in transient recent memory loss for three months, obviously due to stretching of the fornices. In lesions near the trigone of the dominant hemisphere an occipital interhemispheric approach with cortical incision just above the level of the trigone was used[10] in order to avoid damage to the speech centers (Fig. 3). The posterior portion of the third ventricle was exposed by the right occipital interhemispheric transtentorial approach[18].

A temporary external CSF drainage was routinely inserted for several days and this was helpful to avoid permanent shunts in the majority of cases. A two step procedure with CSF diversion prior to tumor operation was only found necessary in cases of extreme hydrocephalus and in emergencies.

Three patients with malignant tumors received postoperative standard radiotherapy, combined with chemotherapy in two.

Results

Following this strategy surgical intervention resulted in complete tumor removal in all patients but one. This was a 4-year-old boy with malignant ependymoma of the third ventricle.

Tumor recurrences were not encountered hitherto although, at least in the cases of malignant ependymoma, a definitive statement is not allowed. There was no operative mortality and operative complications were confined to one subdural hygroma, one chronic subdural hematoma and one subacute epidural hematoma outside the bone flap, which were probably caused by the acute release of raised intracranial pressure during operation. One patient who had not received routine external CSF diversion presented with severe signs of occlusive hydrocephalus a few days later.

Looking at the postoperative morbidity, we encountered two patients with permanent slight hemiparesis, two others with transient hemiparesis and transient hemianopia, respectively, and the above mentioned patient with recent memory impairment for three months.

Discussion

Among the various kinds of intraventricular tumors[5-7, 11, 13, 14, 17, 19-22] there are several which may be identified prior to operation on the basis of age distribution, clinical history and typical CT findings: colloid cysts, epidermoids and teratomas, plexus papillomas, subependymomas and subependymal giant cell astrocytomas[8, 9, 20]. In the present series a preoperative type-specific diagnosis was possible in 6 out of 10 different types of lesions, representing 80% of cases.

Table 1. *Supratentorial Intraventricular Tumors: Clinical Data, CT Findings and Postoperative Outcome*. (Patient no. 16 had multiple tumors: bilateral acoustic neurinomas, small neurinomas of facial and vagal nerves, parasagittal meningeoma, multiple small infratentorial meningeomas, third ventricle meningeoma)

Case no.	Age (years), sex	Histological diagnosis	Location	Signs and symptoms	Type-specific diagnosis by CT	Complications, post-operative morbidity	Follow-up (years)
1	19, m	subepend. giant cell astrocytoma	left frontal	headache, papilledema	yes	slight hemiparesis	9
2	14, f	pineocytoma	post. 3rd v.	headache	no	none	9
3	12, m	teratoma	ant. 3rd v.	headache	yes	CSF accumulat.	8
4	12, f	subepend. giant cell astrocytoma	left frontal	papilledema	yes	none	8
5	12, m	subepend. giant cell astrocytoma	right frontal	sudden onset of coma	yes	chronic subd. hematoma	7
6	2, m	plexus papilloma	right trigone	macrocephaly	yes	none	7
7	17, f	subepend. giant cell astrocytoma	right frontal	seizures, headache	yes	subac. epidural hematoma	6
8	17, f	subepend. giant cell astrocytoma	left frontal	seizures	yes	transient loss of recent memory	6
9	17, m	colloid cyst	ant. 3rd v.	intermittent headache	yes	none	5
10	4/12, m	plexus papilloma	left trigone	asymmetric macrocephaly	yes	transient hemiparesis	4
11	13, m	subependymoma	right frontal	focal seizures, headache	yes	none	4
12	18, f	cavernoma	left frontal	papilledema, psychoorganic syndrome	no	none	3
13	7/12, m	plexus cysts	right trigone	macrocephaly, hemiparesis	yes	none	3
14	14, f	plexus carcinoma	right trigone	headache, diplopia	yes	none	3
15	17, m	subepend. giant cell astrocytoma	right frontal	headache	yes	none	3
16	18, m	meningeoma	ant. 3rd v.	headache	no	none	2 7/12
17	4/12, m	plexus papilloma	ant. 3rd v.	macrocephaly	yes	hygroma, slight hemiparesis	2 6/12
18	9, m	subepend. giant cell astrocytoma	left frontal	headache, mentally retarded	yes	none	2 4/12
19	17, f	subependymoma	left trigone	seizure	yes	transient hemianopia	1 2/12
20	9, f	ependymoblastoma	post. 3rd v.	headache, papilledema	no	none	8/12
21	4, m	ependymoblastoma	ant. 3rd v.	papilledema, hemiparesis	no	none	4/12

Most of these tumors develop within the lateral ventricles. By contrast, many tumors within the third ventricle cannot be differentiated on the basis of clinical data and CT examination[4, 5, 9] and can be identified only by surgical exploration. Moreover, malignancy could be predicted in no case.

Most authors agree about the appropriate surgical approaches to the lateral ventricles[13, 22], apart from the fact that the occipital interhemispheric approach to the trigone of the dominant hemisphere as described by Kempe[10] obviously is rarely used. In our experience a slight modification of this approach proved to be quite satisfactory.

Several authors proposed a variety of approaches to the third ventricle[1-3, 6, 12, 23]; among these the frontal transcallosal approach[1] and the infratentorial supra-

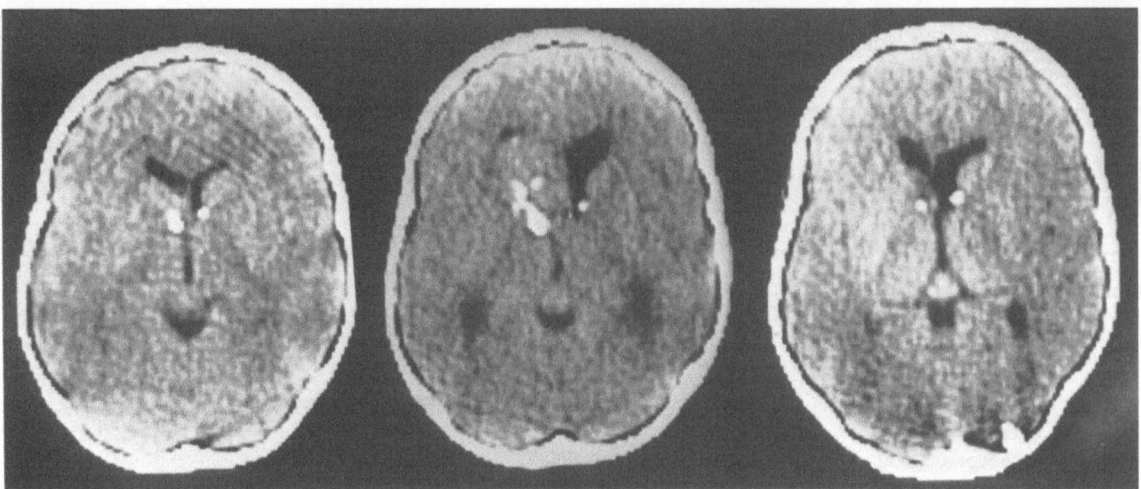

Fig. 2. Case,No. 18. Serial CT scans of a boy, 8 years old at time of operation. Left = 3 years before, middle = just before and right = 1 year after removal of a subependymal giant cell astrocytoma

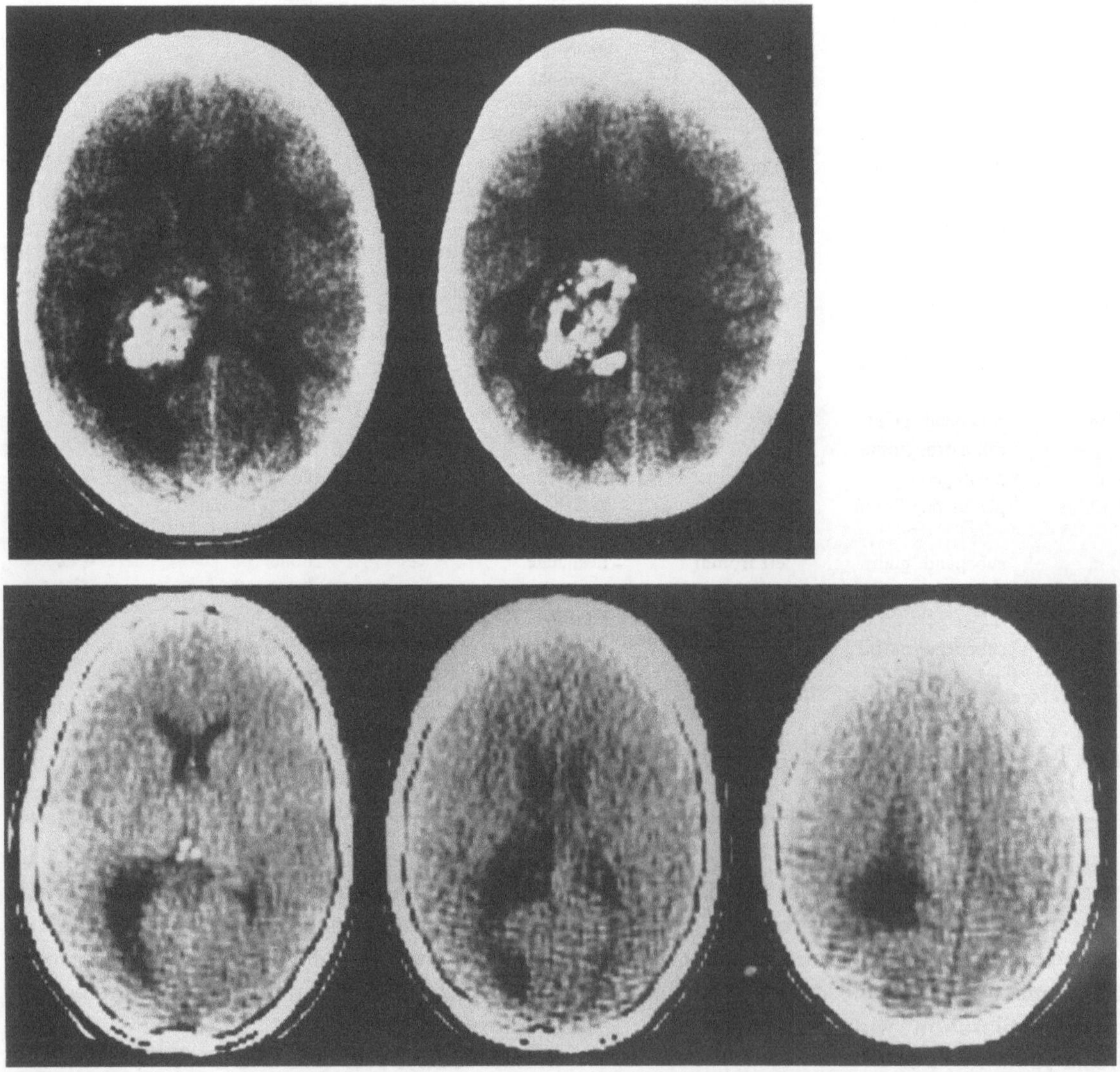

Fig. 3. Case No. 19. Above = before removal of a subependymoma within the left trigone by an occipital interhemispheric approach. Below = 6 months after operation

cerebellar approach[12, 23] have been particularly emphasized. In the present series all lesions within the third ventricle could be sufficiently exposed using the classical routes described by Dandy[2] and Poppen[18]. Surgical treatment is limited in malignant lesions and in tumors invading the ventricular walls and underlying sensitive structures as in case no. 20. Differentiation between paraventricular lesions and intraventricular tumors in the strict sense therefore seems to be justified[11,17].

In conclusion, using an appropriate operative approach based on precise radiological information and meticulous microsurgical technique the majority of ventricular tumors in children and adolescents can be totally removed without severe side effects. Surgical attacks on these lesions no longer carry the high grade of risk which accounted for the emphatic skepticism of former years[25].

References

1. Apuzzo, M. L. J., Chikovani, O. Gott, P., *et al.*, Transcallosal, interfornicial approaches for lesions affecting the third ventricle: surgical considerations and consequences. Neurosurgery *10* (1982), 547–554.
2. Dandy, W. A., Benign Tumors in the Third Ventricle of the Brain: Diagnosis and Treatment. Springfield, Ill.: Ch. C Thomas. 1933.
3. Cossu, M., Lubinu, F., Orunesu, G., Pau, A., Sehrbundt Viale, E., Sini, M. G., Turtas, S.: Subchoroidal approach to the third ventricle. Microsurgical anatomy. Surg. Neurol. *21* (1984), 325–331.
4. Eresue, J., Casenave, P., Guibert Tranier, F. *et al.*, Contribution of radiology to tumors of the third ventricle. J. Neuroradiol. *10* (1983), 345–354.
5. Giromini, D., Pfeiffer, J., Tzonos, T., Über zwei Fälle von Ventrikelmeningeomen im Kindesalter. Neurochirurgia *24* (1981), 144–146.
6. Hoffman, H. H., Transcallosal approach to pineal tumors and the hospital for sick children series of pineal region tumors. In: Diagnosis and Treatment of Pineal Region Tumors (Neuwelt, E.A., ed.). Baltimore-London: Williams and Wilkins. 1984.
7. Jooma, R., Third ventricle choroid plexus papillomas. Childs Brain *10* (1983), 242–250.
8. Kazner, E., Kretzschmar, K., Computer tomographic diagnosis of CNS tumors in childhood. In: Tumors of the Central Nervous System in Infancy and Childhood (Voth, D., *et al.*, eds.), pp. 115–121. Berlin-Heidelberg-New York: Springer. 1982.
9. Kazner, E., Wende, S., Grumme, Th., Lanksch, W., Stochdorph, O., Computed Tomography in Intracranial Tumors. Berlin-Heidelberg-New York: Springer. 1982.
10. Kempe, L. G., Blaylock, R., Lateral trigonal intraventricular tumors. A new operative approach. Acta Neurochir. *35* (1976), 233–242.
11. Koos, W. T., Miller, M. H., Intracranial Tumors of Infants and Children. Stuttgart: Thieme. 1971.
12. Krause, F., Operative Freilegung der Vierhügel, nebst Beobachtungen über Hirndruck und Dekompression. Zbl. Chir. 53 (1926), 2812–2819.
13. Lapras, C., Deruty, R., Bret, Ph., Tumors of the lateral ventricles. In: Advances and Technical Standards in Neurosurgery, Vol. 11 (Krayenbühl, H., *et al.*, eds.). Wien-New York: Springer. 1984.
14. Maspes, P. E., Geuna, E., Resultats du traitement chirurgical de 182 cas de tumeurs du troisième ventricule. Neurochirurgie *12* (1966), 633–636.
15. Masson, C. B., Complete removal of two tumors of the third ventricle with complete recovery. Arch. Surg. *38* (1934), 527–537.
16. Matson, D. D., Neurosurgery in Infancy and Childhood. Springfield, Ill.: Ch. C Thomas. 1969.
17. Pecker, J., Ferrand, B., Javalet, A., Tumeurs du troisième ventricule. Neurochirurgie *12* (1966), 7–136.
18. Poppen, J. L., The right occipital approach to a pinealoma. J. Neurosurg. *25* (1966), 706–710.
19. Poppen, J. L., Marino, R., Pinealomas and tumors of the posterior portion of the third ventricle. J. Neurosurg. *28* (1968), 357–365.
20. Probst, F. P., Erasmie, U., Nergardh, A., Brun, A., CT-appearances of brain lesions in tuberous sclerosis and their morphological basis. Ann. Radiol. *22* (1979), 171–183.
21. Shulman, K., Shapiro, K., Colloid cysts of the third ventricle in infancy and childhood. In: Pediatric Neurosurgery (Section of Pediatric Neurosurgery of the American Association of Neurological Surgeons, ed.), pp. 469–474. New York-London: Grune & Stratton. 1982.
22. Spencer, D. D., Collins, W. F., Surgical management of lateral intraventricular tumors. In: Operative Neurosurgical Techniques, Vol. 1 (Schmidek, H. H., Sweet, W. H., eds.), pp. 561–574. New York-London: Grune & Stratton. 1982.
23. Stein, B. M., The infratentorial supracerebellar approach to pineal lesions. J. Neurosurg. *35* (1971), 197–202.
24. Tsuchida, T., Kamata, K., Kawamata, M., Okada, K., Tanaka, R., Oyake, Y., Brain tumors in tuberous sclerosis. Child's Brain *8* (1981), 271–283.
25. Torkildsen, A., Should extirpation be attempted in cases of neoplasm in or near the third ventricle of the brain? Experiences with a palliative method. J. Neurosurg. *5* (1948), 249–275.

Author's address: Prof. Dr. E. Kazner, Spandauer Damm 130, D-1000 Berlin 19.

Acta Neurochirurgica, Suppl. 35, 80–83 (1985)
© by Springer-Verlag 1985

Primary Cystic Midline Lesions of the Brain in Childhood

St. Comninos, N. Prodromou, and **G. Archondakis**

Department of Neurosurgery, Childrens Hospital "Aghia Sophia", Athens, Greece

Summary

It is known that primary cystic lesions of the midline of the brain in infants and children are not rare.

In some cases these cystic lesions are considered to be the main cause in the production of hydrocephalus. The use of CT-scan tomography and CT scan metrizamide cisternography helped us to reveal some unsuspected cases of them.

Our operative approach of these cystic lesions of the midline of the brain is described.

Keywords: Cyst of the brain; cysts of the midline of the brain.

Cysts of the midline of the brain (excluding tumoral and parasitic cysts) may occur above or below the tentorium, in the tentorial notch or in both intracranial compartments encroaching the tentorium (Anderson et al.[1], Choux et al.[4], Franck et al.[8]).

The cysts contain colorless, CSF-like or slightly xanthochromic fluid: They may be primary located either within cavities preexisting normally in the embryonic life or in potential spaces (cisterns), or may be within the arachnoid formed by closed compartments segregated from the subarachnoid space.

Secondary or leptomeningeal cysts are pockets of the subarachnoid space which are more or less separated from the remainder of the subarachnoid space of adhesions and they may be posttraumatic, postinfective. or posthemorrhagic (Frank et al.[8], Starkman et al.[22]). Cystic lesions of the midline may occur in the locations referred in Table 1. The most common are the cysts of the cisterna magna and the suprasellar arachnoidal cysts.

Material, Methods and Results

In the follow up examination of 500 cases of hydrocephalus which were treated operatively in our

Table 1. *Location of Primary Cysts of the Midline of the Brain in Childhood*

1. Cavum pellucidum
2. Cavum vergae
3. Cavum veli interpositi
4. Tela choroidea
5. Cisterna venae magnae galeni
6. Cisterna quadrigemini
7. Suprasellar arachnoidal cysts
8. Arachnoidal cysts of the cisterna magna
9. Dandy-Walker syndrome

department, for the last ten years we included the CT scan tomography as a routine examination method.

In this clinical material of the last ten years unsuspected cystic lesions of the midline of the brain have been recorded which proved to be the main factor of hydrocephalus and often the cause of the poor results and of repeating attempts of shunting procedures. 22 cases of such cystic lesions of the midline were encountered in our material.

The age of the patients varied from 1 month to 10 years. There was no significant difference in frequency between boys and girls. The location of the cysts is described in Table 2. The most common location was the posterior fossa. The clinical findings and symptoms are shown in Table 3.

The most frequent finding in our material was an enlarged head and hydrocephalus. In older children impaired vision was also a frequent finding. Precocious isosexual puberty was noted in two suprasellar arachnoid cysts and the Bobble-head doll syndrome was noted in a case of a suprasellar cyst and in two cases of Dandy-Walker syndrome.

Table 2. *Location of 22 Cysts of the Midline of the Brain in Infants and Children*

1. Septum pellucidum	(3)
2. Cavum vergae	(1)
3. Cavum veli interpositi	(2)
4. Tela choroidea	(2)
5. Vena magna galeni	(2)
6. Suprasellar	(4)
7. Dandy-Walker	(7)
8. Cisterna magna	(4)

Table 3. *Clinical Symptoms and Findings in Cystic Lesions of the Midline of the Brain*

Infants	Children
1. Enlarged head	1. Headache
2. Hydrocephalus	2. Strabismus
3. Irritability	3. Papilledema
4. Persistent vomiting	4. Impaired vision
5. Convulsions	5. Parinaud's syndrome
6. Generalized weakness	6. Hemianopia
7. Hyperreflexia	7. Bobble-head doll syndrome
8. Failure to thrive	8. Precocious puberty

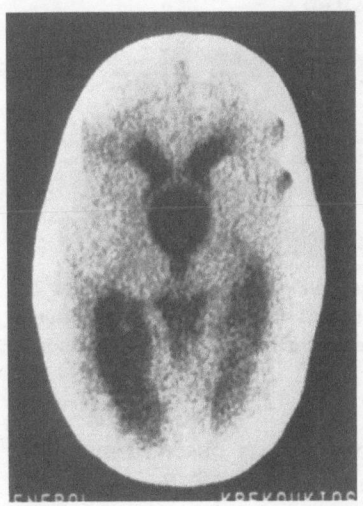

Fig. 1. CT-scan findings in a case of midline archnoidal cyst

Neuroradiological Diagnostic Examinations

CT-scan was in all cases a very helpful examination for establishing the diagnosis. The cystic lesions were clearly demarcated in the CT-scan, non enhancing and showed a globular hypodensity. Cystic neoplasmas could be distinguished by the presence of an enhancing mass and by a thicker surrounding membrane (Banna et al.[2], Schimmel et al.[20]).

In some cases we conducted air studies to make a more accurate localisation of the cyst.

Contrast ventriculography and cystography proved also to be of diagnostic value.

Angiography helped us also in the differential diagnosis of many of the cystic lesions of the midline of the brain, especially of the posterior fossa (Raimondi[18]). Isotope cisternography and more recently metrizamide enhancing CT-cisternography were also of considerable diagnostic value. This has been reported also by Glasauer *et al.*[9], Conway *et al.*[6], Globulof *et al.*[10].

Treatment

In the two cases of cysts of the septum pellucidum with obstruction of the foramen of Monro and hydrocephalus a shunt (V-P) of both ventricles connected by an Y-connector was necessary to control an increased intracranial pressure.

The cystic lesions of the tela choroidea and of the cisterna venae Galeni were of a considerable size and the shunting of the ventricles was not sufficient to control the increased intracranial pressure. A direct surgical approach of the cyst and removal of the cystic wall was necessary to alleviate the symptoms of hypertension.

In the suprasellar arachnoidal cysts the lateral ventricles and the cavity of the cyst were shunted separately. In the majority of the cases it was necessary to drain both lateral ventricles by two different ventricular catheters connected by an Y-connector.

In the cysts of the posterior fossa (cysts of the cisterna magna and cysts of the Dandy-Walker syndrome) it was also necessary to drain the lateral ventricles and the cyst separately and in two cases with two shunt devices of different opening pressure. The results were rather satisfactory (Figs. 1, 2, 3, 4, 5, 6, 7).

Discussion

It is well known that cysts of the septum pellucidum, cavum vergae and veli interpositi are rarely of a size large enough to cause symptoms (Caffey[5]).

In two cases of cysts of the septum pellucidum with hydrocephalus and with obstruction of the foramen of Monro it was, however, necessary to drain the lateral ventricles.

Cysts of the tela choroidea, of the cisterna venae Galeni and of the quadrigeminal plate may reach a considerable size and may be the cause of hydrocephalus and increased intracranial pressure.

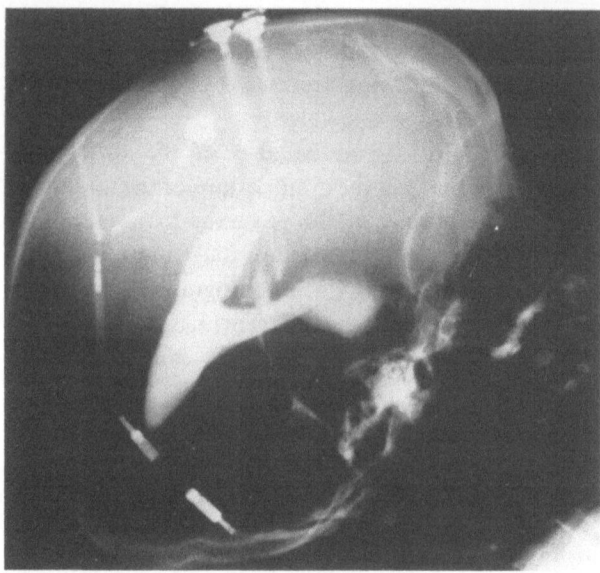

Fig. 2. Same patient as in Fig. 1. Postoperative ventriculogram, showing the communication of the midline cyst with the ventricular system

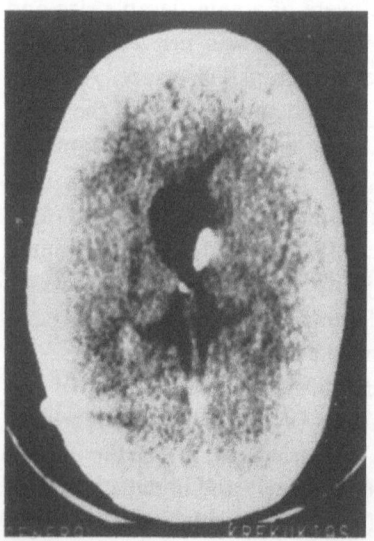

Fig. 3. Postoperative CT-scan in the same patient as of Fig. 1, showing the response of the ventricular system to shunting. The tip of the catheter seems to be located in the cyst

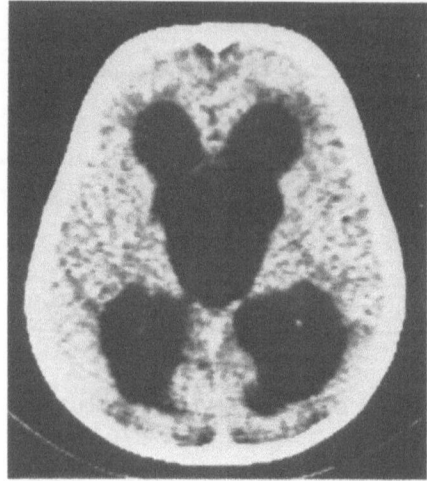

Fig. 4. Preoperative CT-scan in another case of a midline arachnoidal cyst

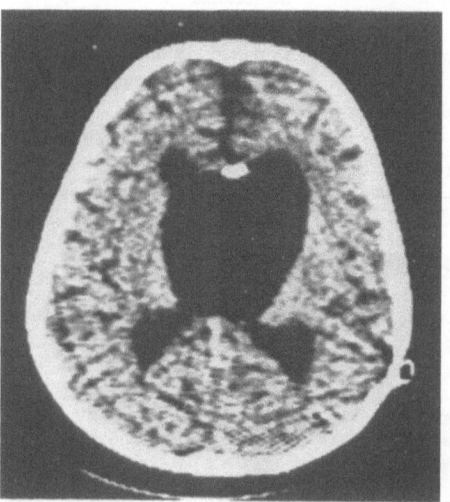

Fig. 5. Postoperative CT-scan in the same patient as in Fig. 4. The reduction in size of one ventricle is shown after shunting. The other ventricle is still dilated, obviously from an obstruction of the foramen of Monro by the cyst

In this case removal of the wall of the cyst to produce a free communication of the cystic cavity with the subarachnoid space will be necessary (Huckman *et al.*[12], Lourie *et al.*[13]).

As it is known, suprasellar arachnoidal cysts are segregated intraarachnoid pockets not communicating usually with the ventricles or with the subarachnoid space. They exercise pressure on the aquaeductus sylvii, the optical pathway and on the hypothalamus. The most striking symptom of hypothalamic dysfunction is the isosexual precocious puberty observed mainly in boys (Farris *et al.*[7], Sansregret *et al.*[19], Segall *et al.*[21]).

A very peculiar symptom encountered in suprasellar arachnoidal cysts is also the bobbing of the head which is described by Benton *et al.*[3], as the Bobble-head doll syndrome (Mayher *et al.*[14], Obenchain *et al.*[15], Patriquin[16]).

Concerning the cysts of the posterior fossa Raimondi *et al.*[17] advocated that craniotomy or either opening of the fourth ventricle into the cisterna magna and third ventriculostomy were of no therapeutic value. They showed that shunt is usually enough, but a shunt should be inserted between the lateral ventricle and the cyst on the one hand and the peritoneum on the other hand in

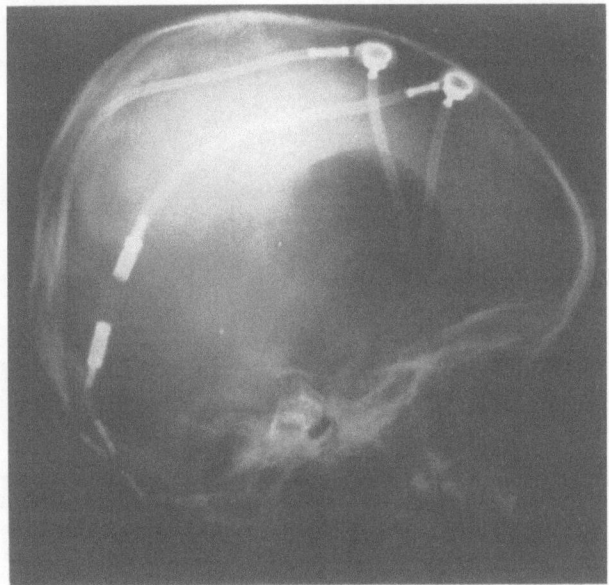

Fig. 6. Same patient as in Figs. 4 and 5. A scond catheter was inserted into the cyst and an air study was carried out, which shows that communication between the cyst and the ventricular system is not existing

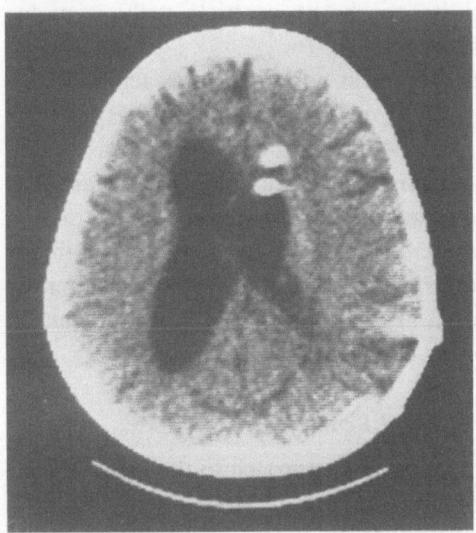

Fig. 7. Same patient as in Fig. 6. After the combined drainage of the ventricles and the arachnoidal cyst, the reduction in size of the ventricular system and of the cyst is obvious

order to avoid a secondary aqueductal occlusion from an upward displacement of the vermis.

On the other hand Hirsch *et al.*[11] supported lately the opinion that the same results can be obtained with a simple cyst-peritoneal shunt.

In our cases of cysts of the posterior fossa it was necessary to shunt separately the ventricles and the cyst, with shunt devices of opening pressure correlated with the pressure inside of the cavity to be drained. The results were mostly satisfactory with no mortality and a very low morbidity rate (20%).

References

1. Anderson, F. M., Landing, B. H., Cerebral arachnoid cysts in infants. J. Pediatr. *69* (1966), 88–96.
2. Banna, M., Arachnoid cysts on computed tomography. Am. J. Roentgenol. *127* (1976), 979–982.
3. Benton, J. M., Nellhaus, G., Hottenlocher, P. R., Ojemann, R. S., Dodge, R. F., The Bobble-head doll syndrome. Neurology (Minneapolis) *16* (1966), 725–729.
4. Choux, M., Raybaud, G., Pinsard, N., Hasson J., Gambarelli, D., Intracranial supratentorial cysts in children excluding tumor and parasitic cysts. Child's Brain *4* (1978), 13–32.
5. Gaffey, J., Pediatric X-Ray Diagnosis, 7th ed., pp. 168-175. St. Louis: Year Book Med. Publ. 1978.
6. Conway, J. J., Yarzagaray, E., Welch, D., Radionuclide evaluation of the Dandy-Walker malformation and congenital arachnoid cysts of the posterior fossa. Am. J. Roentgenolog. Rad. Ther. Nucl. Med. *112* (1971), 306–314.
7. Farris. A. A., Bale, G. F., Cannon, B., Arachnoid cysts of the third ventricle with precocious puberty. S. Afr. Med. J. *64* (1971), 1139–1142.
8. Franck, H., Gruber, M. D., Post-traumatic leptomeningeal cysts. Am. J. Roentgenol. *105* (1969), 305–308.
9. Glasauer, E. F., Isotope cisternography and ventriculography in congenital anomalies of the central nervous system. J. Neurosurg. *43* (1975), 18–25.
10. Goluboff, L. G., Arachnoid cyst of the posterior fossa demonstrated by isotope cisternography. J. Nucl. Med. *14* (1973), 14–61.
11. Hirsch, J. F., Kahn, P., Renier, D., Saint-Rose, Ch., Hoppe-Hirsch, E., The Dandy-Walker malformation. J. Neurosurg. *61* (1984), 515–522.
12. Huckman, M. S., Davis, D. O., Coxe, W. S., Arachnoid cyst of the quadrigeminal plate. Case report. J. Neurosurg. *32* (1970), 367–370.
13. Lourie, H., Berne, S. A., Radiological and clinical features of an arachnoidal cyst of the quadrigeminal plate. J. Neurol. Neurosurg. Psychiat. *24* (1961), 374–378.
14. Mayher, W. F., Gindin, R. A., Head bobbing associated with third ventricular cyst. Arch. Neurol. *32* (1970), 274–277.
15. Obenchain, T. G., Becker, D. P., Head bobbing associated with a cyst of the third ventricle. J. Neurosurg. *37* (1973), 457–459.
16. Patriquin, H. B., The Bobble-head doll syndrome. Radiology *107* (1973), 171–172.
17. Raimondi, A., Samuelsen, G., Yarzagaray, L., Atresis of the foramina of Luschka and Magendie. The Dandy-Walker malformation. J. Neurosurg. *31* (1969), 202–216.
18. Raimondi, A., Pediatric Neuroradiology, 1st ed., pp. 32–65, 168–175. Philadelphia: W. B. Saunders Co. 1972.
19. Sansreget, A., Ledoux, R., Duplantis, F., Lamoureux, C., Suprasellar subarachnoid cysts. Am. J. Roentgenol. *105* (1969), 291–297.
20. Schimmel, D. H., Weinstein, M., Suprasellar subarachnoid cysts. Neuroradiology *II* (1976), 141–146.
21. Segall, H. D., Hassan, G., Ling, S. M., Carton, C., Suprasellar cysts associated with isosexual precocious puberty. Radiology *III* (1974), 607–616.
22. Starkman, S. P, Broun, T. C., Linell, E. A., Cerebral arachnoid cysts. J. Neuropathol. Exp. Neurol. *17* (1958), 484–500.

Author's address: Prof. Dr. Stamatis Comninos, 15 Rizari Street, Athens, Greece.

Acta Neurochirurgica, Suppl. 35, 84–88 (1985)

Possibilities and Limits of the Midline Interhemispheric Approach

J. M. Gilsbach, H. R. Eggert, and **W. Hassler**

Neurochirurgische Universitätsklinik, Albert-Ludwigs-Universität, Freiburg i. Br., Federal Republic of Germany

Summary

Based on experience in 17 children operated upon between 1978 and 1984, the possibilities and limitations of the interhemispheric parafalx approach to lesions of the anterior and posterior lateral ventricles and the third ventricle are described. The interhemispheric approach seems more advantageous than transcortical approaches since additional cortical and white matter lesions can be avoided. The limitations of visibility are the same as in transcortical approaches.

Keywords: Interhemispheric approach; ventricular lesions; trigone; galenic system.

Introduction

The interhemispheric parafalx approach to lesions in the lateral and third ventricles and in the trigone is becoming more and more popular[21, 25, 27]. We prefer this approach whenever possible, especially since we know from investigations among adults that partial sectioning of the corpus callosum does not cause harmful functional deficits[6, 9, 17].

Case Material

Our experience is based on 17 children (Table 1). They were operated on between 1978 and 1984 through an interhemispheric approach under microsurgical conditions. At the same time, 8 children with similar lesions were operated on via a transcortical route. In these cases either the tumor or an enlarged ventricle had reached the cortical surface or a previous operation had left a transcortical defect.

Technique

In deciding on the approach, it is important to make sure that the course and the orifice of the bridging veins do not present a hindrance. For this purpose, we routinely perform angiograms in an oblique view[24].

Nevertheless one or two smaller veins were occluded in 30% of our cases. But neither was a large vein cut, nor did venous infarction occur. Surgery should be done with the patient in a semisitting position and lumbar or ventricular drainage. These are essential to reduce the intracranial volume and pressure. Otherwise it may be very difficult to reach the ventricle without undue spatula pressure.

In all cases we used an unilateral approach through a small parasagittal trepanation, which overlapped the midline by only about 1 centimeter. In contrast to the small bony opening, the medial cortical surface was widely dissected in order to allow tension free retraction of the hemisphere. In lesions located laterally in the ventricle, the corpus callosum was incised 1 cm laterally from the midline after the cingulate gyrus was detached from the corpus callosum (Fig. 1).

Frontal Horn / Third Ventricle

The interhemispheric approach to the frontal horn, the region of the foramen of Monro, and the third ventricle requires that the anterior part of the corpus callosum is incised. But a classical transcortical approach means an additional lesion of the brain substance and partial disconnection of the frontal lobe[17] (Fig. 2). In all of our cases, the working space through the interhemispheric fissure was sufficient. However, it was not always easy to handle lateral tumors in the angle between the corpus callosum and the caudate nucleus. The problems we had with exposure through a narrow foramen of Monro and at the bottom of the third ventricle were not directly associated with the interhemispheric approach but with the lesions themselves. In anterior third ventricle lesions the limits of visibility were reached at the infundibular recess, and a pterional or fronto-basal

Table 1

Patient	Age	Location	Pathology	Approach	Post-operative Complications	Early result
H. S.	12 years	lat. ventr.	giant cell astroc.	interhem.		good
W. B.	16 years	lat. ventr.	giant cell astroc.	interhem.		good
S.	11 years	lat. ventr.	angioma	interhem.	meningitis	good
B. A.	3 years	3rd ventr.	craniopharyngeoma	interhem.	hypoth. dysf.	poor
W. B.	3 years	3rd ventr.	craniopharyngeoma	interhem.	hypoth. dysf.	poor
D. W.	13 years	3rd ventr.	craniopharyngeoma	interhem.	epidural hematoma	fair
M. I.	13 years	3rd ventr.	craniopharyngeoma	interhem.	epidural hematoma	good
W. B.	11 years	3rd ventr.	glioma	interhem.	unchanged	poor
B. D.	4 months	3rd ventr.	plexus papilloma	interhem.		good
W. R.	9 years	3rd ventr.	teratoma	subocc.		good
S. B.	13 years	3rd ventr.	germinoma	subocc.	meningitis	poor
K. A.	13 years	3rd ventr.	hypophyseal tu.	pterional	hypoth. dysf.	fair
V. T.	2 years	trigonum	plexus papilloma	interhem.		good
K. S.	4 months	trigonum	plexus papilloma	transcort.		good
K. D.	9 months	trigonum	plexus papilloma	transcort.		good
H. S.	9 years	basal gangl.	angioma	interhem.		good
K. M.	14 years	basal gangl.	angioma	interhem.	hydrocephalus	fair
K. M.	15 years	basal gangl.	angioma	transcort.		fair
S. C.	3 weeks	galenic syst.	angioma	interhem.		failed
B. A.	12 days	galenic syst.	angioma	interhem.	hemorrhage	poor
B. A.	4 months	galenic syst.	angioma	interhem.	hemorrhage	poor
S. M.	7 months	galenic syst.	angioma	interhem.		good
M. S.	9 months	galenic syst.	angioma	interhem.		good
K. S.	10 months	galenic syst.	angioma	subtemp.		good
G. K.	2 years	galenic syst.	angioma	subtemp.	+ electrothromb.	good

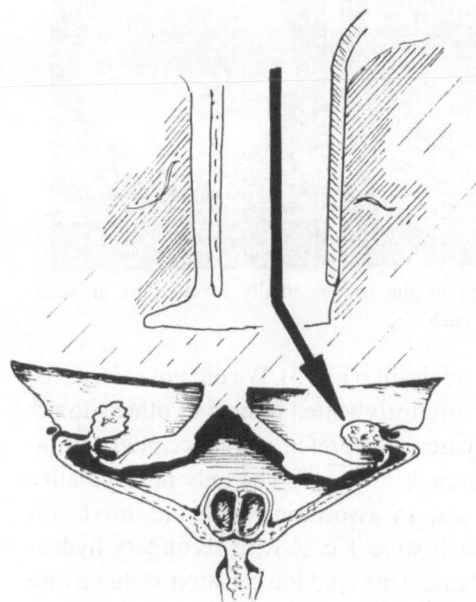

Fig. 1. For lesions located laterally in the ventricle, the incision in the corpus callosum is made as lateral as possible after the cingulate gyrus is dissected *

* Figs. 1, 2, 3, and 5 by courtesy of Prof. Seeger and Springer-Verlag Wien-New York.

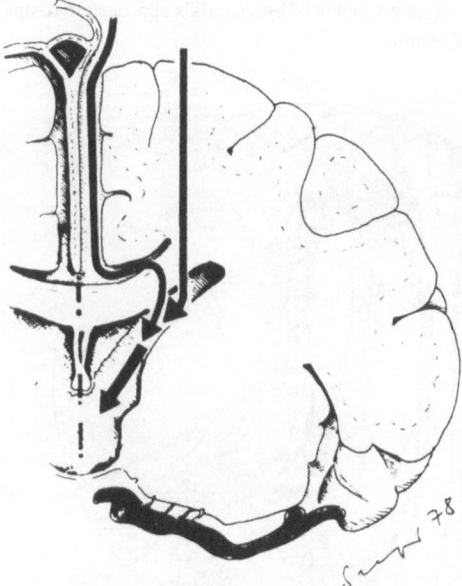

Fig. 2. The incision of the corpus callosum in a parafalx and transcortical approach is nearly the same but the latter involves an additional brain lesion *

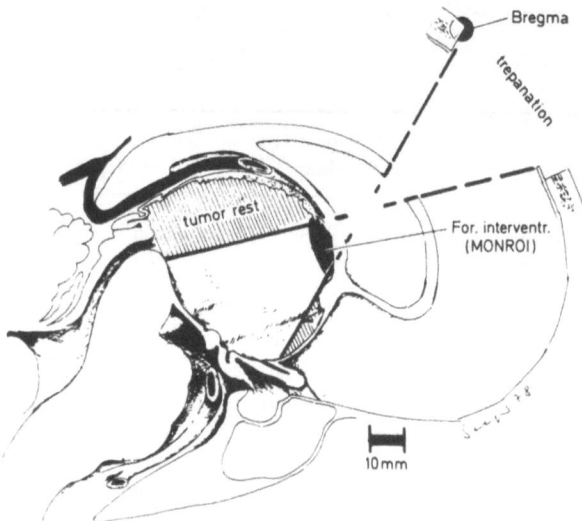

Fig. 3. The anterior and dorsal part of the third ventricle cannot be seen entirely from a parafalx approach without damaging the anterior border of the foramen Monro (fornix) *

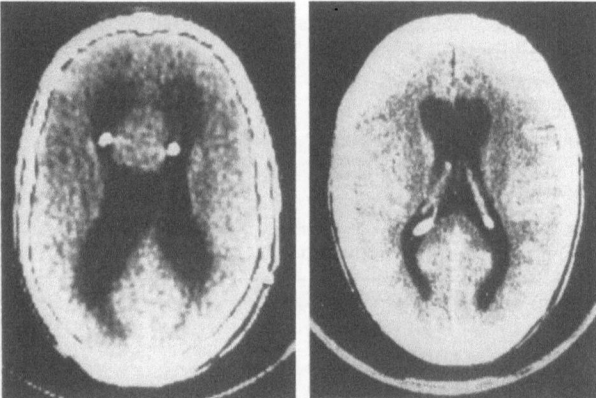

Fig. 4. Typical case of a giant cell astrocytoma in the lateral ventricle (frontal horn), which was removed by a parafalx approach to re-open the foramen of Monro

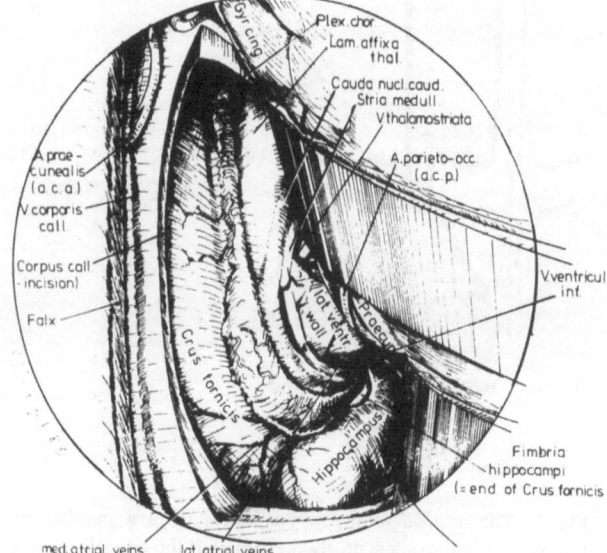

Fig. 5. View of the trigone from a parafalx approach in the region of the precuneus through the incised splenium *

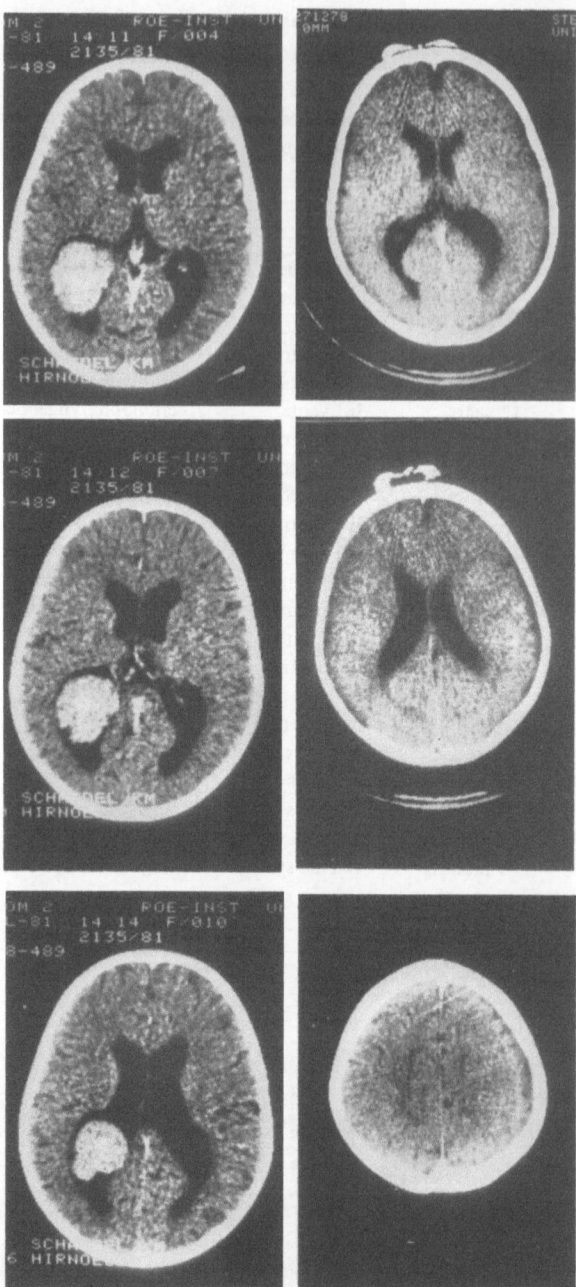

Fig. 6. Papilloma of the trigone totally removed by an inter-hemispheric approach

approach was advisable (Fig. 3). We did not enlarge the foramen for posteriorly seated tumors as others do[2, 13, 30]. In these cases we prefer a suboccipital supra-cerebellar approach[18, 20, 22, 26]. The only postoperative problems we saw in association with the interhemi-spheric approach were 1 case with secondary hydro-cephalus and 2 cases with epidural hematomas. In no case did a transcortical approach seem more advantageous (Fig. 4).

Trigone

Interhemispheric approaches to the trigone have rarely been described[5, 11, 14]. More popular is the

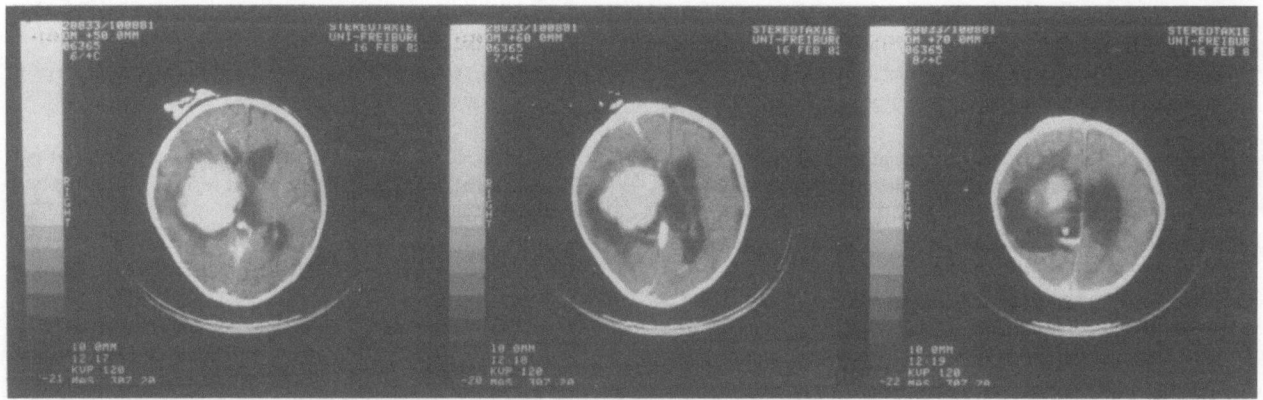

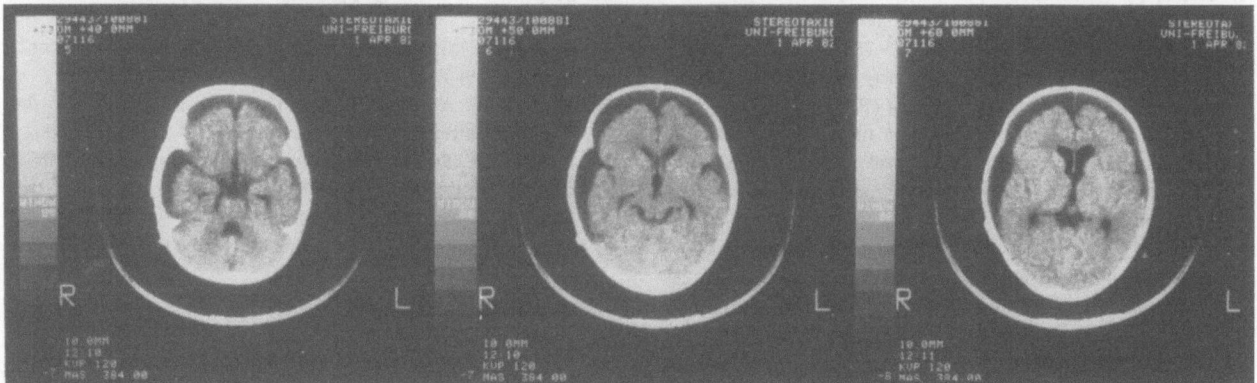

Fig. 7. In this case of a trigonal tumor in which a cyst or the enlarged ventricle reached the cortical surface, a direct transcortical approach was preferable

transcortical route through a parietal[3, 5], parieto-occipital[7, 10, 15, 16, 19, 29] or temporal gyrus[4, 7, 8, 10, 12, 16, 28, 31]. We use the interhemispheric route parallel to the precuneus with splitting of the distal third of the corpus callosum (Fig. 5). However, we preserve the splenium because a totally disrupted splenium may cause major deficits[17]. The one child with a medium-sized papilloma tolerated the operation without any deficits, especially without visual disturbances (Fig. 6). But the lateral parts of the tumor, which were directed towards the temporal horn, were at the limits of accessibility. In such cases it may be necessary to partially resect the fusiform or cingulate gyrus[27]. The results were also satisfactory in 2 cases in which a transcortial route was considered better because a cyst or the tumor itself was seated just below the cortex (Fig. 7).

Galenic System

Five A.V. malformations of the Galenic system were approached through a unilateral parieto-occipital parafalx route[1, 32]. In one case of a three-week-old child we failed to open the interhemispheric fissure because of raised intracranial pressure. As an alternative treatment, stereotactically inserted wires were used to induce thrombosis. Two other children were operated on subtemporally. In only one case, in which large subdural effusions provided enough room for exposure, were we able to remove the angioma.

Conclusions

The interhemispheric approach to the lateral ventricle including the trigone is practicable, safe, and without unnecessary morbidity. One minor disadvantage is the limited lateral visibility. The visibility and accessibility of lesions in the third ventricle depend not only on the approach but on the anatomical situation. The least traumatic approach, namely the interhemispheric approach, is therefore preferable.

References

1. Amacher, A. L., Shillito, J., The syndroms and surgical treatment of aneurysms of the great vein of Galen. J. Neurosurg. *39* (1973), 89–98.

2. Apuzzo, M. L. J., Chikovani, O. K., Gott, P. S., Teng, E. L., Zee, C. S., Giannotta, S. L., Weiss, M. H., Transcallosal, interfornical approaches for lesions affecting the third ventricle: surgical consideration and consequences. Neurosurgery *10* (1982), 547–554.

3. Cramer, F., The intraventricular meningiomas: a note on the neurologic determinants governing the surgical approach. Arch. Neurol.*3* (1960), 98–99.

4. Delandsheer, J. M., Les meningiomes du ventricule lateral. Neurochirurgie *11* (1965), 3–57.

5. Fornari, M., Savoiardo, M., Morello, G., Solero, C. L., Meningiomas of the lateral ventricles. Neuroradiological and surgical considerations in 18 cases. J. Neurosurg. *54* (1981), 64–74.

6. Geffen, G., Walsh, A., Simpson, D., Jeeves, M., Comparison of the effects of transcortical and transcallosal removal of intraventricular tumors. Brain *103* (1980), 773–788.

7. Guidetti, B., Spallone, A., The surgical treatment of choroid plexus papillomas. Neurosurg. Rev. *4* (1981), 129–137.

8. Hoffman, H. J., Supratentorial brain tumors in children. In: Neurological Surgery, Vol. 5 (Youmans, J. R., ed.), pp. 2702–2732. Philadelphia-London-Toronto-Mexico City-Sydney-Tokyo: Saunders. 1982.

9. Jeeves, M. A., Simpson, D. A., Geffen, G., Functional consequences of the transcallosal removal of intraventricular tumors. J. Neurol., Neurosurg., Psychiatr. *42* (1979), 134–142.

10. Kempe, L. G., Operative Neurosurgery. Berlin-Heidelberg-New York: Springer. 1968.

11. Kempe, L. G., Blaylock, R., Lateral-trigonal intraventricular tumors. A new operative approach. Acta Neurochir. *35* (1976), 233–242.

12. Laurence, K. M., The biology of choroid plexus papilloma and carcinoma of the lateral ventricle. In: Handbook of Clinical Neurology. Vol. 17 (Vinken, P. J. Bruyn, G. W., eds.), Amsterdam: North-Holland. 1974.

13. Lavyne, M. H., Patterson, R. H., Subchoroidal trans-velum interpositum approach to mid-third ventricular tumors. Neurosurgery *12* (1983), 86–94.

14. Levin, H. S., Rose, J. E., Alexia without agraphia in a musician after transcallosal removal of a left intraventricular meningioma. Neurosurgery *4* (1979), 168–174.

15. MacCarty, C. S., Piepgras, D. G., Ebersold, M. J., Meningeal tumors of the brain. In: Neurological Surgery, Vol. 5 (Youmans, J. R., ed.), pp. 2936–2966. Philadelphia-London-Toronto-Mexico City-Sydney-Tokyo: Saunders. 1982.

16. Matson, D. D., Crofton, F. D. L., Papilloma of the choroid plexus in childhood. J. Neurosurg. *17* (1960), 1002–1027.

17. Oepen, G., Schulz-Weiling, R., Zimmermann, P., Birg, W., Stresser, S., Gilsbach, J., Long term effects of partial callosal lesions. Acta Neurochir., in publication.

18. Page, L. K., The infratentorial-supracerebellar exposure of tumors in the pineal area. Neurosurgery *1* (1977), 36–40.

19. Raimondi, A. J., Gutierrez, F. A., Diagnosis and surgical treatment of choroid plexus papillomas. Child's Brain *1* (1975), 81–115.

20. Reid, W. S., Clark, W. K., Comparison of the intratentorial and transtentorial approaches to the pineal region. Neurosurgery *3* (1978), 1–8.

21. Rhoton, A. L., Yamamoto, I., Peace, D. A., Microsurgery of the third ventricle, part 2: operative approaches. Neurosurgery *8* (1981), 357–373

22. Sano, K., Matsutani, M., Pinealoma (germinoma) treated by direct surgery and postoperative irradiation. Child's Brain *8* (1981), 81–97.

23. Seeger, W., Microsurgery of the Brain. Wien-New York: Springer. 1980.

24. Seeger, W., Microsurgery of Cerebral Veins. Wien-New York: Springer. 1984.

25. Shucart, W. A., Stein, B. M., Transcallosal approach to the anterior ventricular system. Neurosurgery *3* (1978), 339–343.

26. Stein, B. M., Supracerebellar-infratentorial approach to pineal tumors. Surg. Neurol. *11* (1979), 331–337.

27. Stein, B. M., Arteriovenous malformations of the medial cerebral hemisphere and the limbic system. J. Neurosurg. *60* (1984), 23–31.

28. de la Torre, E., Alexander, E., jr., Davis, Ch., jr., *et al.*, Tumors of the lateral ventricles of the brain: report of eight cases with suggestions for clinical management. J. Neurosurg. *20* (1963), 461–470.

29. Turcotte, J. F., Copty, M., Bedard, F., Michaud, J., Verret, S., Lateral ventricle choroid plexus papilloma and communicating hydrocephalus. Surg. Neurol. *13* (1980), 143–146.

30. Viale, G. L., Turtas, S., The subchoroid approach to the third ventricle. Surg. Neurol. *14* (1980), 71–76.

31. Walsh, L., Supratentorial intraventricular tumors. In: Operative surgery (Symon, L., ed.), pp.174–180. London-Boston: Butterworths. 1979.

32. Yaşargil, M. G., Antic, J., Laciga, R., Jain, K. K., Boone, S. C., Arteriovenous malformations of vein of Galen. Microsurgical treatment. Surg. Neurol. *6* (1976), 195–200.

Author's address: Joachim M. Gilsbach, M.D.*, Hans R. Eggert, M.D., Werner Hassler, M.D., Neurochirurgische Klinik, Universität Freiburg, Hugstetter Strasse 55, D-7800 Freiburg i. Br., Federal Republic of Germany.

* Request for reprints.

Acta Neurochirurgica, Suppl. 35, 89–91 (1985)

Surgical Treatment of Intraventricular Meningiomas in Childhood

M. Mircevski, D. Mircevska, I. Bojadziev, and **R. Basevska**

Clinic for Surgical Diseases, Section of Pediatric Neurosurgery, University of "Cyril and Methody", Skopje, Yugoslavia

Summary

In the last ten years (1973–1983) we operated and followed up 6 patients with intraventricular meningiomas, of these 4 were children and 2 adults.

In 3 of the children the meningiomas occupied the lateral ventricles and were attached to the choroid plexus and the medial brain structures. The fourth childhood tumor was localized in the posterior third of the third ventricle. The first three children were operated by the established procedure for ventricular tumors, while the fourth was subjected to the procedure of Cl. Lapras (Lyon, France) for meningiomas and other tumors in the posterior part of the third ventricle.

All four children survived the procedure. In the follow-up period they showed normal mental and physical development.

Keywords: Intraventricular meningiomas; localization; surgical treatment.

Introduction

Intracranial meningiomas are quite rare in childhood. In the majority of published papers their incidence is reported to be 1–2% of all intracranial tumors. Intraventricular meningiomas are more common in children than in adults[3, 4, 5, 10].

According to some authors (Merten *et al.*; Gori and Nucci) they account for 15–17%[4] of all intracranial meningiomas. In our material their incidence was 14%. We thought that a report on our 4 children with intraventricular meningiomas would be of interest, because in 2 of them the diagnosis was made before the advent of CT scanning and in the remaining 2 after CT had become available[7, 8]. In particular, we would like to draw attention to the case with intraventricular meningioma in the posterior third of the third ventricle[5, 7, 8].

Clinical Material and Methods

Within a period of ten years (1973–1983) we operated and followed up 4 children with intraventricular meningiomas. Three of these involved the lateral ventricles and were attached to the choroid plexus, while one occupied the posterior third of the third ventricle. The sex distribution was 3 males versus 1 female. Patient age was 8, 11, 15, and 16 years (Table 1).

Table 1. *Localization of Intraventricular Meningiomas*

Region	Number of cases
Right parietal horn of lateral ventricle	1
Right occipital horn of lateral ventricle	1
Left occipital horn of lateral ventricle	1
Posterior third of third ventricle	1

For a long time before the diagnosis can be made intraventricular meningiomas are asymptomatic. Grand mal seizures and headaches were among the first symptoms followed by loss of vision. In the later stage of the disease all the children developed hydrocephalus. All four children were admitted as emergency cases with changes in consciousness, stupor, somnolence and incipient incarceration.

The oldest child (age 16 years) had well developed muscles because of weight lifting (Fig. 1). He was soporous on admission, but regained consciousness after antiedematous therapy for subsequent surgery. The diagnosis was based on the history and physical examination, plain skull X-rays, EEG, CT, gamma encephalography and arteriography. In the 2 children undergoing CT the diagnosis was no problem. But in the other two arteriography and gamma encephalography had to be repeated. They showed the typical signs of intraventricular expansion. The definitve diagnosis was confirmed by the histopathology of the surgical specimens.

Surgical Treatment

Ventriculoperitoneal drainage was instituted in 2 children because of the hydrocephalus, the other 2

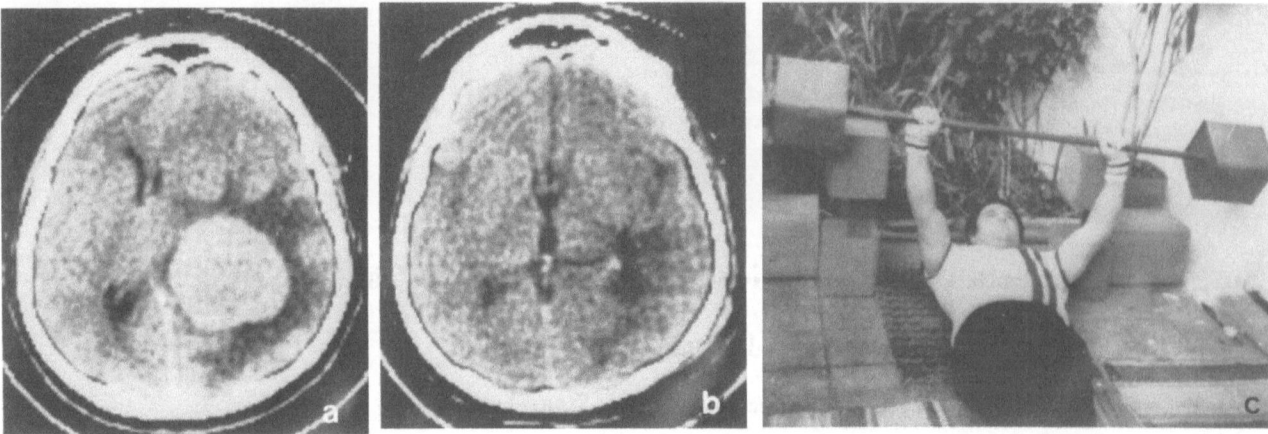

Fig. 1. 16-year-old child with right occipital intraventricular mass lesion. CT-Scan before (a) and after (b) operation. Patient six months after surgery (c)

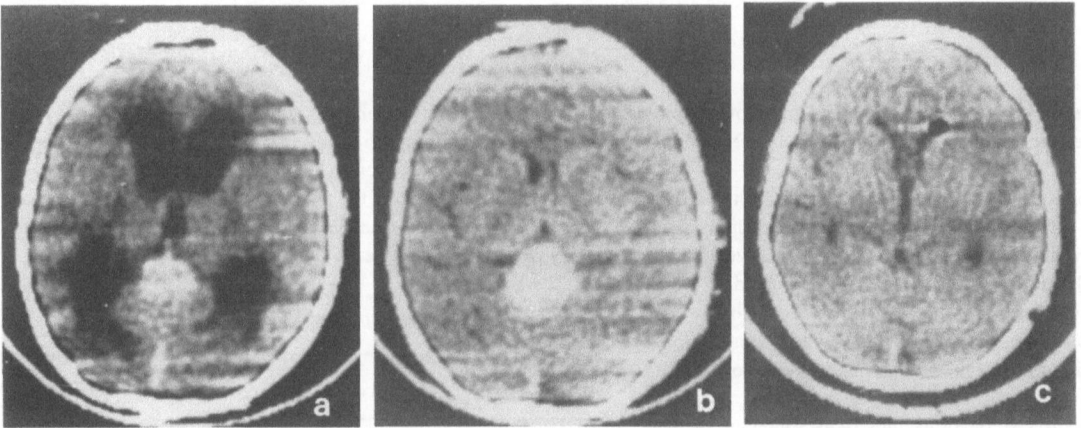

Fig. 2. 11-year-old child with a mass lesion in the posterior third of the third ventricle with hydrocephalus (a) and after shunting procedure (b). CT-Scan control three months after radical operation according to Lapras (c)

received antiedematous therapy (20% manitol and dexamethason, 4 mg). After recovering from their comatose state they were operated in a relatively stable condition. Surgery consisted in craniotomy and the approach normally used for ventricular tumors in the parietal and occipital horns has to be shortly defined. There do exist several possibilities. In two tumors localized in the occipital horns, the access consisted in a corticotomy in the parieto-occipital region and opening of the ventricle where the tumor was locateds, while in the third case a corticotomy was performed. In the frontal region slightly backwards towards temporo-parietal and the frontal horn was opened and finally the tumor was localized beneath and backwards of the foramen of Monro. A special approach was chosen in the forth case (Fig. 2). With the child sitting, parietooc-cipital craniotomy was done in the midline and the dura/tentorium cerebelli were opened bilaterally, great care being taken to spare the major vessels. This brought into view the pineal region and the posterior third of the third ventricle. With this special method described by Claude Lapras from Lyon adequate access was obtained for extirpating the tumor which was as big as a large egg.

All four tumors were extirpated totally. They turned out to be meningiomas of the haemangioblastic type.

Results

All 4 children survived treatment. Shunts were removed in the post-operative follow-up period since the hydrocephalus had disappeared or did no longer manifest itself. Within 6 months to 1 year the children returned to normal life.

Since the oldest child (age 16 years) was obese and had an excessive muscle mass, we put him on a diet with acceptable improvement within 5 years. His mental and emotional problems also improved within one year.

The other children were asymptomatic throughout the follow-up period of 2 to 10 years.

Discussion

Intraventricular tumors, especially meningiomas, are extremely rare tumors of the central nervous system. They account for 1–2% of all the intracranial meningiomas in children and adults. Some authors postulated a predominance of females and the left temporal ventricle[3, 4, 5, 9, 10]. Before the CT era they were hardly ever diagnosed pre-operatively. This is why patients were admitted in a comatose, stuporous or somnolent state, produced by the concomitant hydrocephalus.

The key methods for diagnosis were arteriography and ventriculography. On arteriography the choroidal artery was the "master" sign. It was readily visualized in one of our cases. In two cases we had good diagnostic results with gamma encephalography.

Since CT was introduced in 1978 the diagnosis has been established immediately after admission. Confirmation was obtained with the other diagnostic procedures.

The definitive diagnosis of meningiomas is histological. In all four cases, the haemangioblastic component dominated the histological picture, other components were endothelial, fibroblastic and typically angiomatous. The operative technique, including that of Claude Lapras for tumors in the posterior third of the third ventricle, provides for adequate radicality, while sparing the surrounding structures. This ensures survival without sequels. During the procedure we were sure of the diagnosis and the radicality of the extirpation, the latter being confirmed by post-operative CT[4, 5, 11] There was no need for radiotherapy or other adjuvant treatment modalities. During surgery careful dissection and preservation of the major vessels surrounding the meningioma are critically important. Care should be taken to dissect the afferent vessels first before turning to the efferent ones[1, 3, 5, 6]. Our results support the concept that ventricular meningiomas can and should be operated even if they are localized in the posterior third of the third ventricle.

References

1. Cooper, M., Dohn, D. F., Intracranial meningiomas in childhood. Cleve. Clinic. *41* (1974), 197–204.
2. Cushing, H. W., Eisenhard, L., Meningiomas, their Classification, Regional Behaviour, Life History and Surgical Results. Springfield, Ill., U.S.A.: Ch. C Thomas. 1938.
3. Gassel, M. M., Davies, H., Meningiomas in the lateral ventricle. Brain *84* (1961), 605–627.
4. Gori, G., Nucci, V., Meningeomi dell'infanzia e dell'eta evolutiva. Considerazione statistiche e cliniche. Minerva Neurochir. *7*, 119–124.
5. Lapras, Cl., Personal Communication, 1972, 1983, 1984.
6. Leibel, S. A., Wara, W. M., Sheline, G. E., Townsed, J. J., Boldrey, E. B., Treatment of meningiomas in childhood. Cancer *37* (1976), 2709–2712.
7. Mircevski, M., Basevska, R., Dzonov, I., Mircevska, D., Méningiomes cérébraux de localisation et d'évolution clinique particulières. 33e Congrès de la Société de Neurochirurgie de Langue Française Marrakech, Morocco, May 5, 6, 7, 1983.
8. Mircevski, M., Basevska, R., Ruskov, P., Davkov, S., Mircevska, D., Surgical Treatment of CNS Meningiomas with specific localization and evolution. 20 years of the Society of Polish Neurosurgery Warsaw, October 19–21, 1984.
9. Mendiratta, S. S., Rosenblum, J. A., Strobos, R. J., Congenital meningioma. Neurology *17* (1967), 914–917.
10. Russel, D. S., Rubinstein, L. J., Pathology of Tumours of the Nervous System. London: Edward Arnold Ltd. 1977.
11. Koos, W. Th., Miller, M. H., Intracranial Tumours of Infants and Children, pp. 118–124. Stuttgart: Thieme. 1971.

Author's addresses: Dr. M. Mircevski, Ivan Cankar 28, Vlae, 91000 Skopje, Yugoslavia, Dr. Danica Mircevska, Ivan Cankar 28,Vlae, 91000 Skopje, Yugoslavia, Dr. Ilija Bojadziev, Clinic for Children's Diseases, Medical Faculty, Vodnjanska 17, 91000 Skopje, Yugoslavia, and Dr. Roza Basevska, Department of Anesthesiology, Clinic of Surgical Diseases, Medical Faculty, 91000 Skopje, Yugoslavia.

Acta Neurochirurgica, Suppl. 35, 92–93 (1985)

Supratentorial Astrocytomas of the Midline in Childhood—
A Review of Treatment and Prognosis

H. Pothe

Department of Neurosurgery, Medical Academy of Erfurt, German Democratic Republic

Summary

Supratentorial astrocytomas in childhood are rare. In our series of 47 children (1979–1983) suffering from intracerebral tumors we observed three with astrocytomas situated in the midline. They had invaded the walls of the ventricles and caused hydrocephalus. The children were operated on by a right transventricular approach. We succeeded in total tumor removal in two cases and these children are well. One child (only subtotal extirpation had been possible) died. In our opinion, resignation is unfounded in such cases.

Keywords: Astrocytoma; childhood; Midline; Results of treatment.

Introduction

Supratentorial astrocytomas in childhood are relatively rare[2]. This is especially true for those located in the midline. Our interest in this localisation is derived from the tendency of these tumors to compress the third ventricle or the foramina of Monro. Compression results in an obstruction of the CSF pathways and leads to the development of hydrocephalus.

Astrocytomas in this topographical area are seldom true tumors of the third ventricle. The latter, by definition, arise from or fill the ventricular cavity. In terms of this definition astrocytomas are, in reality, commonly extraaxial and extraventricular tumors encroaching upon the ventricle walls.

Although their incidence is low their surgical management constitutes a formidable challenge for the neurosurgeon[1] because of the anatomical situation of the third ventricle and the cerebrospinal pathways as well as the relation of the tumor to vital neural structures and hidden deep veins.

Refined methods of diagnosis and treatment necessitated reevaluation of neurosurgical management and prognosis. In light of this, the term "inoperable" will have to be redefined.

Methods and Material

Three tumours out of a series of 47 children suffering from supratentorial intracerebral tumours, which were fare observed during the past five years were located in the midline of the brain. They had invaded the walls of the ventricles, occluding the third ventricle and the pathways of cerebrospinal fluid. The children were operated on by a right transventricular approach. Total removal of the tumors was possible in two cases. Microsurgical techniques were, of course, indispensable.

Case Reports and Results

Case 1: An 8-year-old boy was admitted with the diagnosis of a tumor in the region of the third ventricle (4×5 cm in diameter) compressing both lateral ventricles. He complained of severe episodes of headaches. Bilateral shunting was performed as a first step. Three weeks later the child was operated on by a right transventricular approach. Total extirpation was impossible. The boy died four days after surgery. Autopsy showed that astrocytoma II and III had invaded the midbrain.

Case 2: The first symptom was progressive clumsiness of the right hand in a 12-year-old girl. She was admitted to a neurological service. CT led to the diagnosis of a posterior third ventricular tumor. We succeeded in extirpation of what turned out to be astrocytoma I.

Case 3: A 12-year-old boy complained of slight clumsiness of the left foot for which an orthopedist prescribed a special boot. Two years later the parents observed incidental vomiting. Computed tomography showed a solid tumor in the third ventricle compressing the lateral ventricles (Figs. 1 and 2). With a right transventricular approach total extirpation of what was a pilocytic astrocytoma I was possible and the boy is well (Figs. 3 and 4).

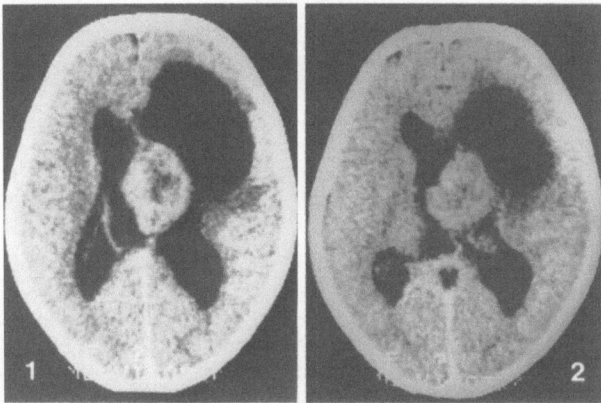

Figs. 1 and 2. Pilocytic astrocytoma in the midline (case 3). Preoperative situation at two different levels

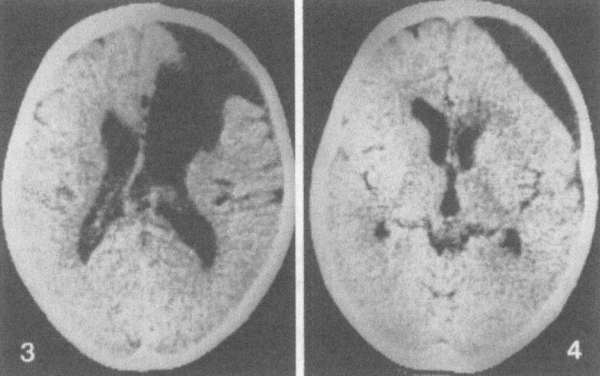

Figs. 3 and 4. Follow-up two months after operation (case 3), same levels as Figs. 1 and 2

Discussion

Among the clinical symptoms headaches and palsies are most prominent in such cases. Computed to-

mography is the examination of choice. Thanks to the differences in density between the tumor tissue, the normal brain and the ventricular fluid diagnosis is easy. Ventriculography with Amipaque is, no doubt, a reliable method, but unnecessary in most cases. Pneumencephalography may be dangerous because of potentially raised intracranial pressure.

In most of the publications on the subject the majority of space-occupying midline lesions are thought to be ineligible for total surgical removal. Often shunt procedures are advocated.

Nevertheless our position is to operate on all of these tumors. After all, the introduction of the operative microscope has greatly facilitated the exposure of this hidden area. Whenever total removal is ruled out, biopsy will, as a rule, be absolutely necessary for rational and directed radiotherapy.

References

1. Isamat, F., Tumors of the third ventricle. Fourth postgraduate course in neurosurgery. Montpellier: La Grande Motte. 1977.
2. Jänisch, W., Güthert, H.,. Schreiber, D., Pathologie der Tumoren des Zentralnervensystems, 1. Auflage, S. 189–202. Jena: G. Fischer 1976.

Author's address: Prof. Dr. Dr. H. Pothe, Department of Neurosurgery, Surgical Clinic, Medical Academy of Erfurt, Nordhäuser Strasse 74, DDR-5010 Erfurt, German Democratic Republic.

Acta Neurochirurgica, Suppl. 35, 94–100 (1985)

G. Sella

Microsurgical Topography of Craniopharyngiomas

J. Šteňo

Department of Neurosurgery, Comenius University, Bratislava, Czechoslovakia

Summary

The relationship of craniopharyngiomas to surrounding structures was studied by stereoscopic and light microscopy in 30 autopsies. The localization of 4 of the tumors was intra- and suprasellar, 26 lesions were primarily suprasellar. Suprasellar craniopharyngiomas were divided into three groups according to their relationship to the floor of the third ventricle: extraventricular[4], intra extraventricular[14] and intraventricular[8]. The different localization of craniopharyngiomas in the vertical axis is a codeterminant of the direction and extent of tumor growth in the horizontal plane at the base of the brain. Comparison of these anatomical data and additional anatomical findings obtained in primary microsurgical operations of another 16 patients with the results of plain X-ray and contrast studies revealed radiological features characteristic of different topographic groups. The choice of the most adequate approach and degree of radicality of surgery for craniopharyngiomas can be based on the results of pre-operative neuroradiological investigations.

Keywords: Craniopharyngioma; microsurgical topography; third ventricle.

Introduction

The relationships of craniopharyngiomas to surrounding anatomical structures are characteristically quite variable. The location of the tumor may, therefore, be determined by its relation to different structures of the base of the brain and skull. Present-day topographic classifications of craniopharyngiomas are based on the relationship of the tumor to the sella turcica and the optic chiasm[2, 10, 13]. Quite a large number of craniopharyngiomas is in close contact with hypothalamic structures located in the floor and the walls of the third ventricle, which often precludes safe radical surgery of these benign tumors[7, 8, 15]. Their topographic relationships are not sufficiently clear in the literature. While it is almost generally accepted that nearly all craniopharyngiomas initially grow under the floor of the third ventricle[3, 6, 11, 16] there are rare reports indicating that most craniopharyngiomas[5] develop intracerebrally as intrinsic parts of the infundibulum or tuber from the very outset[12].

The purpose of our study was to establish the topographical relationship of craniopharyngiomas to the floor and the walls of the third ventricle. We also tried to define the delineation of the tumors versus different anatomical structures. Another purpose of our study was to show how these relationships can be determined before the operation by means of neuro-radiological studies.

Material and Methods

The relationships of craniopharyngiomas to surrounding structures were studied in 30 autopsy cases. These had been patients of the Neurosurgical Institutes in Moscow, Kiev, and Leningrad, USSR, and of the Neurosurgical Department in Bratislava, Czecho-slovakia. They had died in the course of a ten-year period (1969–1978) at the ages of 6 to 59; 10 of them were under 15 years of age. In 11 patients the tumor was not attacked directly and in 19 cases it was removed partially, with 5 of these 19 tumors requiring repeated operations.

The brain was removed in the usual manner (22 cases) or together with the dura and the central, perisellar part of the base of the skull (8 cases). The undissected brain (15 cases) or serial sagittal or coronal sections 10 millimeters thick were examined under the stereoscopic microscope, using 5 to 72 fold magnification. Selected specimens were studied by the microtrachiscopic method[1] and by common histological technique.

Detailed anatomical data as well as additional anatomical findings obtained in primary microsurgical operations of another 16

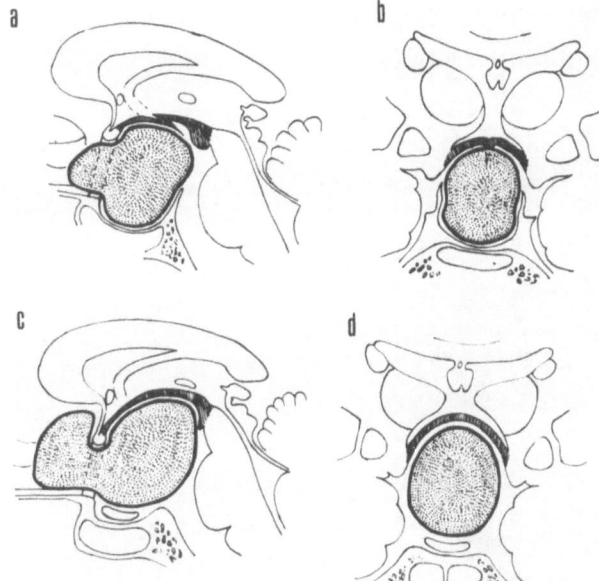

Fig. 1. Relationship of intrasuprasellar (a, b) and suprasellar extraventricular (c, d) craniopharyngiomas to the floor (cross-hatched) and the walls of the third ventricle

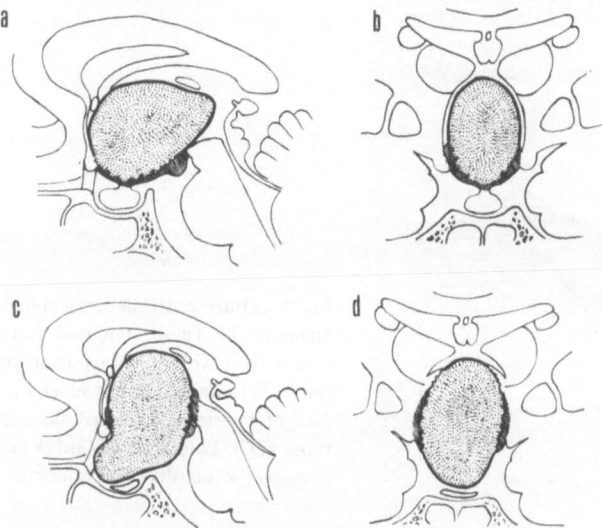

Fig 2. Relationship of intraventricular (a, b) and intra-extraventricular (c, d) craniopharyngiomas to the floor (cross-hatched) and the walls of the third ventricle

patients with craniopharyngiomas operated during the past five years at the ages of 4 to 60 (2 of them under 15 years) were compared with the results of neuroradiological investigations in each case. Pneumo-encephalography and/or ventriculography were performed in 36, carotid angiography in 16 and vertebral angiography in 7 patients. CT scans were available of the last 7 operated patients.

Results

1. Relationship of Craniopharyngiomas to the Third Ventricle

The location of 4 of the tumors of the autopsy series (Table 1) was intra- and suprasellar (Figs. 1 a and b). The thick fibrous capsule of the suprasellar part of what usually was a cystic tumor was separated from the superiorly displaced floor of the third ventricle by an arachnoid membrane. Firm adherence of the tumor capsule to the infundibular region was observed in one unoperated case. In the operative series (Table 1), however, the whole suprasellar part of the tumor could be safely removed in all four patients.

Twenty-six craniopharyngiomas were situated entirely above the sellar diaphragm, *i.e.*, they were primarily suprasellar. Three types of relationships of the tumor to the floor of the ventricle were found. Accordingly, suprasellar craniopharyngiomas were divided into 3 groups: extraventricular, intraventricular and intra- extraventricular.

Extraventricular suprasellar tumors (Figs. 1 c and d) were located in the subarachnoid space. Their superior surface was always connected with the pial membrane of the superiorly displaced ventricular floor by means of fine connective tissue adhesions. By gentle traction the tumor could be detached from the thinned floor of the ventricle without damaging it. This was also the case in the single operation involving an extraventricular suprasellar tumor. Firm adhesions precluding safe removal of the tumor capsule were found only in patients autopsied after repeated operations.

Craniopharyngiomas wholly or partially located in the cavity of the third ventricle (intraventricular or intra-extraventricular craniopharyngiomas) made direct contact with brain tissue.

Table 1. *Topographic Groups of Craniopharyngiomas*

Series	Intrasuprasellar	Suprasellar			Total
		Extraventricular	Intraventricular	Intra-extra-ventricular	
Autopsy	4	4	8	14	30
Operation	4	1	4	7	16

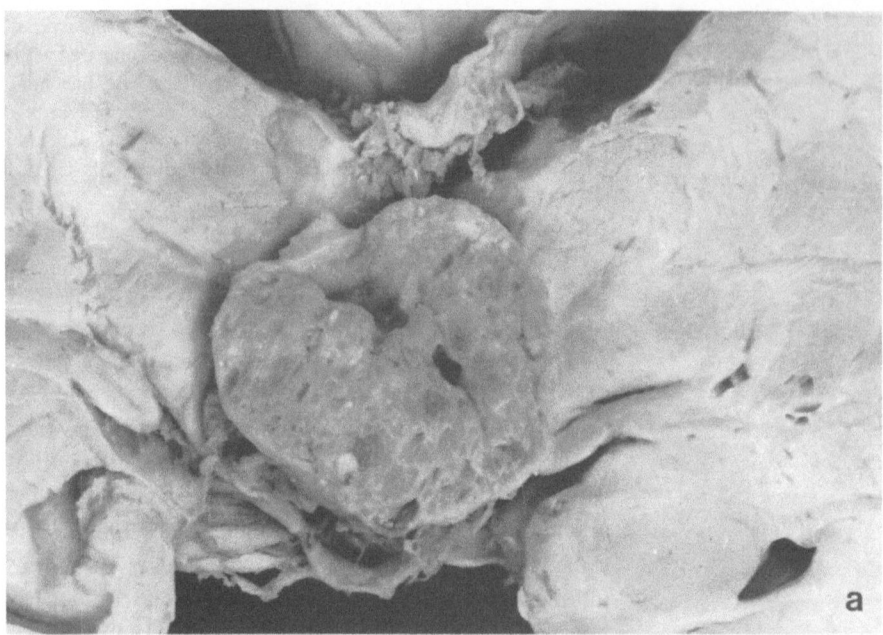

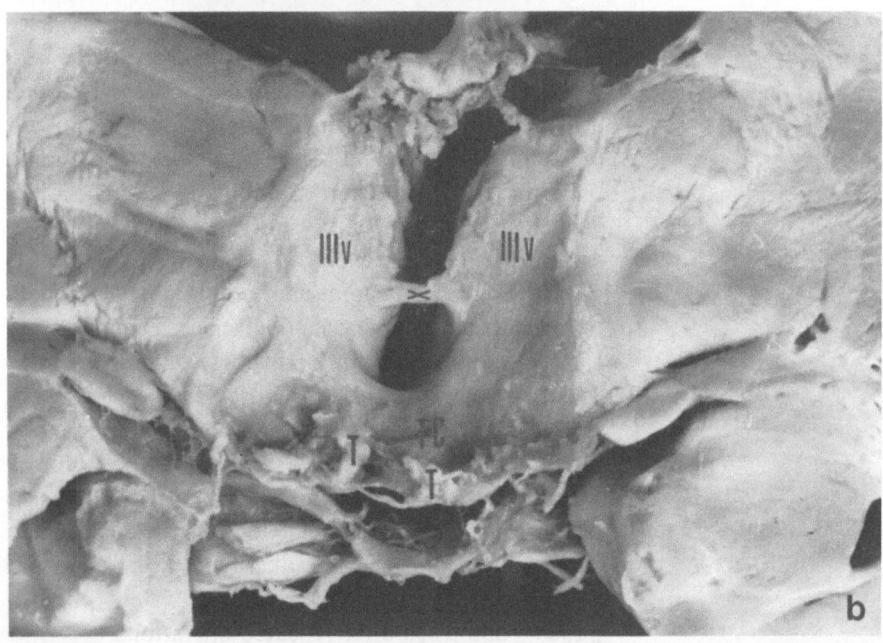

Fig. 3. a) Intraventricular craniopharyngioma; b) Tumor removed from ventricular cavity. Small remnants of tumor (*T*) attached to the inner surface of inferiorly displaced thinned tuber (*TC*). Lateral walls (3rd *v*) undamaged; *x* interthalamic adhesion

In intraventricular craniopharyngiomas the floor of the third ventricle covered the inferior surface of the tumor (Figs. 2 a and b). The brain tissue of the infundibulum and the median part of the tuber showed signs of gliosis and was devoid of nerve cells. Moreover, part of these structures had undergone full atrophy in all cases, so that a small area of the tumor surface was covered with pial membrane only. Well-preserved brain tissue containing normally appearing neurons was found in the lateral parts of the tuber and in the undamaged mammillary bodies.

The gliotic tumor capsule invariably adhered to the remnants of the infundibulum and tuber, in 3 cases it was also attached to the lateral walls of the ventricle. Glial fibrils of brain tissue continued into the depth of the tumor capsule. In 5 cases the lateral aspects of the tumor were wholly or predominantely separated from the ventricular walls lined by ependyma (Fig. 3). Keeping this in mind, we left the basal part of the tumor intact during surgical removal through the foramen of Monro in all 4 patients. The capsule of the larger dorsal part of the tumor was removed only if it was not adherent to the ventricular walls.

In one case a small cystic part of the tumor bulged

downward into the retrosellar region below the level of the ventricular floor. This case represents a transitional form overlapping with the next topographic group of intra-extraventricular craniopharyngiomas.

The remnants of the floor of the third ventricle in intra-extraventricular craniopharyngiomas are situated along the "equator" of the tumor, dividing its dorsal intraventricular portion from a basal extraventricular one (Figs. 2 c and d). Grossly compressed mammillary bodies covered the posterior pole of the tumor. The remnants of the lateral parts of the tuber were situated on the lateral surface of the tumor (Fig. 4). The anterior part of the floor was represented by a band of glial tissue covering the anterior pole of the tumor or, more often, had undergone full atrophy.

A continuation of the pial membrane from the remnants of the floor down to the surface of the extraventricular part of the tumor could be traced in 12 cases. In 8 of them the pia was disrupted at the site of contact of the tumor with the chiasm. Full disruption of the pia mater along the whole tumor-hypothalamus and tumor-chiasm junction was only seen twice. Together with the remnants of the floor and lateral ventricular walls the gliotic capsule of the intraventricular part of the tumor, often a multilocular cyst, formed a single layer of tissue (Fig. 4). Inspite of this the tumor capsule could often be macroscopically detached from the brain without problems but microscopy showed disruption of marginal glial tissue and blood vessels coursing from the brain tissue to the tumor. These vessels were usually small, but in 2 cases their diameter reached 0.1–0.15 millimeters. Moreover, bands of glial tissue about half to one millimeter thick from the lateral ventricular walls continued between the cysts into the depth of the tumor in 2 cases. In another case a cyst 10 millimeters in size growing out of the main tumor mass spread into the lateral hypothalamus.

In 5 out of 7 patients operated on for intra-extraventricular craniopharyngiomas we removed the tumor only partially or subtotally from the third ventricular cavity, leaving adherent portions of tumor tissue in place. One of our 2 radical operations was followed by the only death in the whole series. The patient died one month after the operation from severe hypothalamic disorders.

2. Extension of Craniopharyngiomas in the Horizontal Plane at the Base of the Brain

Extensive anterior growth of the tumor in front of the optic chiasm was observed only in craniopharyngiomas located under the floor of the third ventricle,

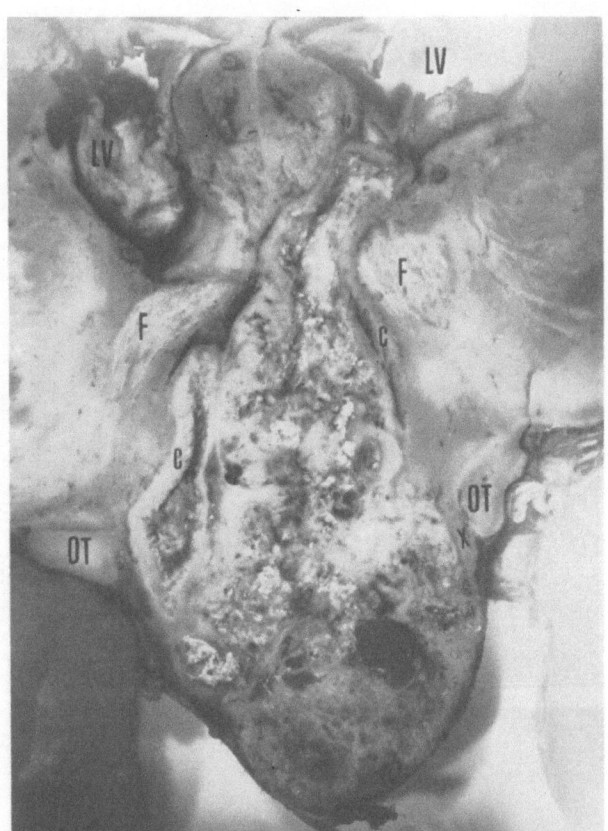

Fig. 4. Intra-extraventricular craniopharyngioma extending into lateral ventricles (*LV*). Tumor capsule (*C*) intimately adheres to lateral walls of the ventricle and to remnants of tuber (*x*). *OT* optic tract; *F* fornix

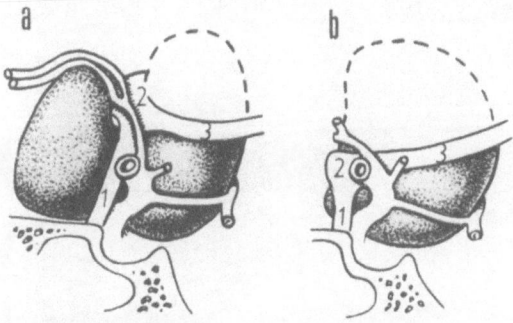

Fig. 5. Relationship of extraventricular (a) and intraextraventricular (b) craniopharyngiomas to optic nerves (*1*), chiasm (*2*) and tracts (*3*) and to the vessels of circle of Willis

i.e., in intra- and suprasellar and extraventricular suprasellar masses (Fig. 5). Rarely extraventricular craniopharyngiomas grew completely behind the chiasm, while retrochiasmal spread was the rule in intra-extraventricular tumors. In cases with congenitally short optic nerves the chiasm was situated on the

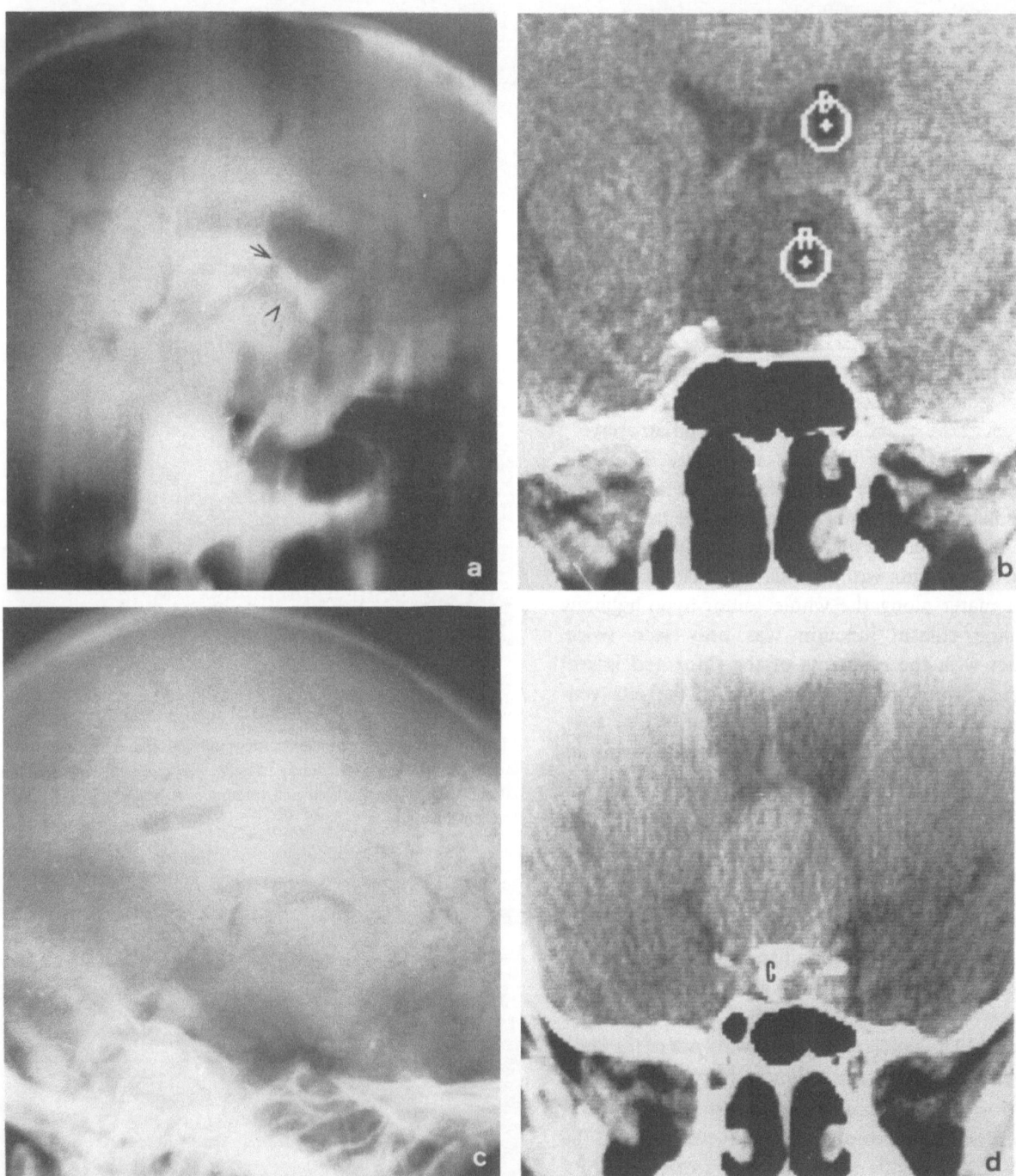

Fig. 6. a) Anterior part of third ventricular cavity (arrowheads) displaced superiorly and anteriorly from foramina of Monro (arrow) by extraventricular suprasellar craniopharyngiomas. "J" shaped sella; b) Tumor-free anterior part of the third ventricle displaced superiorly by extraventricular suprasellar tumor; c) Intraventricular craniopharyngioma; d) Calcified basal portion (C) of intra-extraventricular craniopharyngioma projecting in the anterior part of sellar cavity. Anterior part of the ventricle entirely filled by tumor

inferior anterior aspect of the tumor thus limiting accessibility of the extraventricular part of the tumor by the subchiasmatic approach.

Retrosellar growth was more extensive in suprasellar extraventricular, or intra-extraventricular, versus intra-suprasellar tumors.

Parasellar spread was seen in six cases of different groups. Through the space between the optic tract and the posterior communicating artery the tumor extended towards the temporal lobe and into the Sylvian fissure; in 3 cases it encroached upon the frontal and/or temporal lobes. This mostly cystic part of the tumor often enveloped arteries at the base of the brain. The cyst wall only slightly adhered to major blood vessels, to their branches and to brain structures and could be easily separated in previously unoperated cases.

3. Comparison of Anatomical Data with Results of Neuroradiological Investigation

Tumors growing under the floor of the third ventricle often displaced the anterior part of the ventricular cavity not only upwards but also anteriorly from the foramina of Monro (Figs. 6 a and b). Craniopharyngiomas fully or partially located in the ventricular cavity usually filled its anterior portion entirely so it could not be seen either on lateral pneumograms or on direct coronal CT scans (Figs. 6 c and d). The contour of the filling defect of the ventricle sometimes delineated the lobulated surface of the tumor. Intraventricular tumors caused slight or moderate depression of the "roof" of the suprasellar cisterns, while intra-extraventricular tumors in all but one case precluded filling of the chiasmal cistern and depressed the intercrural, sometimes even the pontine cisterns.

Characteristic "ballooning" of the sella seen on plain roentgenograms distinguished intra-suprasellar from suprasellar craniopharyngiomas, which encroached upon the sella from above. Extraventricular tumors and especially the calcified basal part of intra-extraventricular tumors often extended into the sella displacing its diaphragm downwards. Though in fact suprasellar, the tumor in nearly half of the cases projected into the entrance, or inside the cavity of the sella (Fig. 6 d). This was usually accompanied by gross shortening of the dorsum and marked depression of the tuberculum sellae (Fig. 6 a).

Anterior and posterior extension of craniopharyngiomas was seen on carotid and vertebral angiography, respectively. CT clearly defines all directions of growth and the entire extent of solid and cystic portions of the tumor including its parasellar spread. Especially parasellar cysts enveloping major arteries without displacing them significantly may not be well defined on angiography.

Discussion

The relationship of primarily suprasellar craniopharyngiomas to the floor of the third ventricle and to the meninges found in our series are in disagreement with almost universally accepted concepts about the origin of these tumors under the ventricular floor[3, 6, 11, 16]. Subventricular development was seen in only a minority of primarily suprasellar tumors, namely in extraventricular craniopharyngiomas situated in the subarachnoid space under the ventricular floor with undamaged pial membrane. Characteristic displacement of hypothalamic structures along the "equator" of intra-extraventricular craniopharyngiomas together with a retrochiasmal tumor location supports the concept that their origin is in the depth of the ventricular floor in the infundibular region[5]. Intracerebral development was seen in cases where the pial membrane of the remnants of the ventricular floor and the optic chiasm continued to the basal surface of the tumor. Only in cases where the pia mater was disrupted along part or, exceptionally, the whole boundaries between the intra- and extraventricular portions of the tumor, the concept of a primary infraventricular development and later penetration into the cavity of the ventricle is acceptable.

The position of hypothalamic structures of a partially atrophied ventricular floor on the inferior surface of intraventricular tumors may suggest a derivation from embryonal epithelial remnants in more dorsal subependymal layers of the infundibulum or tuber[14]. After breaking through the subependymal layer and ependyma of the ventricular floor in an early stage of its development the tumor grows freely in the ventricular cavity. This may explain the less intimate relationships of intraventricular craniopharyngiomas to hypothalamic structures compared to intra-extraventricular tumors, although a transitional type of tumor location between these two topographic groups does exist.

Anatomically proven integrity of the third ventricular floor in intraventricular craniopharyngioma is rare[4, 14]. Inspite of the fact that this was never seen in any of our intraventricular tumors, we consider it of practical value to set aside these craniopharyngiomas as a separate group. By characteristic neuroradiological signs it is possible to identify the position of hypothalamic structures attached to the inferior surface of the tumor and avoid their damage during surgery by approaching the tumor through the foramina of Monro, corpus callosum or by opening the lamina terminalis and leaving the basal portion of the tumor intact.

Pre-operative neuroradiological investigations enable us also to distinguish suprasellar extraventricular from intra-extraventricular craniopharyngiomas with a high degree of probability. Different relationships of these tumors to hypothalamic structures require different surgical approaches. The loose connection of extraventricular craniopharyngiomas to the pial membrane of the superiorly displaced thinned ventricular floor and its sufficient exposure under the chiasm usually allow total removal of the tumor. In intra-extraventricular craniopharyngiomas only the extraventricular part of the tumor can be removed radically either from under the chiasm or, in patients with short optic nerves, by opening the lamina terminalis. The intraventricular part of the tumor is firmly embedded in the brain tissue of the hypothalamus. Moreover, a distinction of the tumor from brain tissue is sometimes impossible inspite of using a surgical microscope[8,9]. It is advisable, therefore, to remove only those parts of the tumor which are not adherent to the walls of the third ventricle, as a more radical removal may result in severe damage of the hypothalamus.

References

1. Baron, M. A., Reactive structures of internal membranes (in russ.). Medicina (Leningrad) *1949*, 432–435.
2. Benes, V., Notes on the surgical treatment of craniopharyngiomas (in czech.). Csl. Neurol. *25* (1962), 305–312.
3. van der Bergh, R., Brucher, J. M., L'abord transventriculaire dans les cranio-pharyngiomes du troisième ventricule. Neuro-Chirurgie (Paris) *16* (1970), 51–65.
4. Cashion, E. L., Young, J. M., Intraventricular craniopharyngioma. Report of two cases. J. Neurosurg. *34* (1971), 84–87.
5. Grekhov, V. V., Topography of craniopharyngiomas (in russ.). Vopr. Neirokhir. *23/6* (1959), 12–17.
6. Hoffman, H. J., Hendrick, E. B., Humphreys, R. P., Buncic, J. R., Armstrong, D. L., Jenkin, R. D. T., Management of craniopharyngiomas in children. J. Neurosurg. *47* (1977), 218–227.
7. Ivkov, M., Ribaric, I., Slavik, E., Antunovic, V., Samarzic, M., Djordjevic M., Surgical treatment of craniopharyngiomas in adults. Acta Neurochir. Suppl. *28* (1979), 352–356.
8. Konovalov, A. N., Krasnova, T. S., Microneurosurgical technics in removal of craniopharyngiomas (in russ.). In: The 2nd Congress of Neurosurgery of USSR/Thesea, pp. 201–203. Moscow: 1976
9. Koos, W. Th., Böck, F. W., Pendl, G., Salah, S., Microsurgery of craniopharyngiomas. In: Clinical Microneurosurgery (russ. transl.) (Koos., W.Th., *et al.*, eds.), pp. 52–60. Moscow: Medicina. 1980.
10. Koos, W. Th., Miller, M. H., Intracranial Tumors of Infants and Children, pp. 188–213. Stuttgart: Thieme. 1971.
11. Matson, D. D., Neurosurgery in Infancy and Childhood, 2nd ed., pp. 544–574. Springfield, Ill., U.S.A.: Ch. C Thomas. 1969.
12. Northfield, D. W. C., Rathke-pouch tumors. Brain *105* (1957), 293–323.
13. Rougerie, J., Craniopharyngiomes. Indications thérapeutiques et resultats. Gaz. Med. Fr. *80* (1973), 5225–5232.
14. Schmidt, B., Gherardi, R., Pirier, J., Caron, J. P., Craniopharyngiome pédicule du troisième ventricule. Rev. Neurol. (Paris) *140* (1984), 281–283.
15. Stroobant, C., Evrard, Ph., Belpasire, M. C., Thauvoy, Ch., Ferriere, G., La traitement des craniopharyngiomes intraventriculaires. Acta Neurol. Belg. *75* (1975), 116.
16. Zülch, K. J., Atlas of Gross Neurosurgical Pathology, pp. 155–160. Berlin-Heidelberg-New York: Springer. 1975.

Author's address: J. Šteňo, M.D., Department of Neurosurgery, Comenius University, Limbova 5, 833 05 Bratislava, Czechoslovakia.

Acta Neurochirurgica, Suppl. 35, 101–105 (1985)

Neurosurgical Treatment of Cushing's Disease in Children and Adolescents

M. Buchfelder and **R. Fahlbusch**

Department of Neurosurgery, University of Erlangen-Nürnberg, Federal Republic of Germany

Summary

The authors report on 15 unselected consecutive children and adolescents treated for hypothalamo-pituitary Cushing's disease by transsphenoidal sella exploration and microadenomectomy. The diagnosis was established by dynamic endocrine testing. Peri- and post-operative measurements of ACTH levels were used to monitor the effectivity of the surgical procedure. In one patient no micro-adenoma was found. Hypercortisolism was corrected in 13 of the 15 patients. Although transient secondary adrenocortical insufficiency occurred in all of the successfully operated patients, no permanent damage of the anterior or posterior pituitary was found by post-operative endocrinological follow-up testing. One patient died of pneumonia as a direct consequence of surgery.

Keywords: Cushing's disease; transsphenoidal surgery; selective adenomectomy; hypercortisolism; ACTH; pituitary microadenoma.

Introduction

In a series of 102 patients suffering from Cushing's disease we[4] could, like other authors[1, 6, 7, 14, 16], document that selective adenomectomy of ACTH-secreting microadenomas of the pituitary can eliminate the ACTH excess and restore anterior pituitary function. This seems to be of special importance in childhood since the majority of our young patients had hypopituitarism leading to severe disturbances of development, *i.e.* delayed puberty and impaired growth. Furthermore, the untoward effects of other therapeutic approaches like life-long dependency on corticosteroid substitution following bilateral adrenalectomy should be avoided.

Patients and Methods

This series consists of 15 consecutive unselected patients with onset of the clinical symptoms of Cushing's disease between the age of 7 and 14 years. At the time of the operation they were between 13 and 16 years old (mean age, 14.5 years). Four of the patients were male, 11 were female (Table 1). All of them were operated between 1978 and 1984 in Munich or Erlangen by R.F.

Weight gain (15/15 = 100%), growth retardation (12/15 = 80%) and delayed puberty (11/15 = 73%) were the most common presenting symptoms.

The diagnosis of central ACTH-dependent Cushing's disease was established on the basis of dynamic endocrine testing. To rule out other causes of Cushing's syndrome, we looked for:

1. elevated plasma cortisol levels without circadian rhythm;
2. insufficient suppression of basal cortisol levels after 2 mg of dexamethasone overnight (normal $< 2 \mu g/dl$);
3. at least 50% suppression of plasma cortisol levels after 8 mg dexamethasone;
4. ACTH levels within the normal range (20–50 pg/ml) or only elevated slightly;
5. stimulation of cortisol and ACTH levels by lysine-vasopressine acting like corticotropin releasing hormone (CRH) or by CRH itself.

In addition, all patients underwent routine pre- and post-operative testing of anterior pituitary function[2,15].

All of the patients had plain skull X-rays and sellar polytomograms of 2 mm intervals. Sellar size was found to be normal in all of the patients on plain skull X-rays. A slight pathological bulging of the sellar floor was found in 4 patients by polytomography only. Five patients operated on in Erlangen had thin collimation CT scans with sagittal and coronal reconstructions. In three of these, microadenomas were identified as clear-cut hypodense intrasellar lesions.

The surgical procedure was carried out via a sublabial-paraseptal-transsphenoidal approach thus preserving the patient's nasal mucosa in order not to disturb later nasal growth.

Thin sectioning of the pituitary body was done in order not to miss parts of the tumor. No alcoholic solution was used within the tumor bed. There never was subtotal hypophysectomy or resection of periadenomatous tissue.

Results

Operative Findings

On microsurgical exploration of the pituitary body microadenomas were found in all of the 15 patients

Table 1. *Clinical Data on the 15 Patients with Juvenile Cushing's Disease. In Patient A. B. no Adenoma was Detected. Patient M. H. Died After an Endocrinologically Successful Surgical Procedure* (m = male, f = female, y = years, p = primary amenorrhea, S = secondary amenorrhea)

Patient	Sex	Age onset	Age (year) operation	Prim./Sec. amenorrhea	Delayed puberty	Growth retardation	Clinical outcome
A. B.	m	11 years	14 years (1979)	0	+	+	failure
E. B.	f	9 years	15 years (1979)	P	+	+	remission
M. H.	m	7 years	16 years (1982)	0	+	+	(rem.) died
P. H.	f	12 years	14 years (1980)	S			remission
B. K.	f	12 years	14 years (1980)	P	+	+	remission
A. M.	f	12 years ?	14 years (1980)	P	+	+	remission
J. M.	f	14 years ?	16 years (1983)	S			remission
C. R.	f	11 years	13 years (1984)	P	+		remission
D. S.	f	11 years	15 years (1984)	P	+	+	remission
S. S.	f	10 years	14 years (1979)	P	+	+	remission
M. S.	f	11 years	13 years (1978)	P	+	+	remission
H. W.	f	12 years	13 years (1984)	S		+	remission
W. W.	m	11 years ?	16 years (1980)	0	+	+	remission
G. Z.	m	13 years	16 years (1983)	0	+	+	failure
K. Z.	f	13 years ?	15 years (1981)	S	+		remission

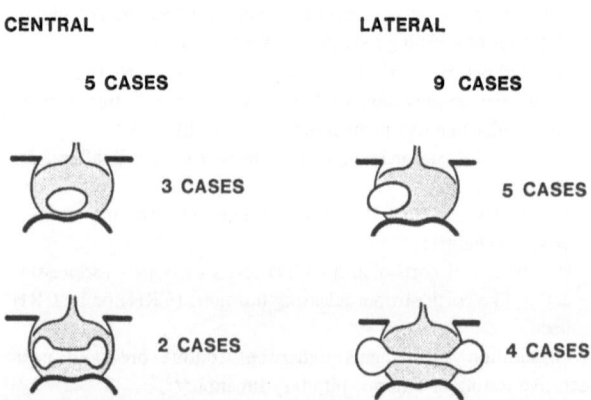

CENTRAL

5 CASES

3 CASES

2 CASES

LATERAL

9 CASES

5 CASES

4 CASES

Fig. 1. Localization of microadenomas found during surgery in 14 patients with juvenile Cushing's disease

with one exception. Fig. 1 demonstrates the localization of these adenomas, five of them being centralized. Three of these central tumors were well circumscribed, the other 2 were more or less diffuse, dumbbell-shaped or surrounded by a pseudocapsule. The majority of the adenomas showed not only intrasellar, but also extraglandular extension, they were lateralized. Again, many had poorly defined outlines. Histological examination by conventional staining revealed a pituitary adenoma in 10 of the patients; 2 had follicular hyperplasia. In 10 cases ACTH secretion could be found by immunehistology or cell culture studies.

Endocrinological Results

In addition to the clinical remission of symptoms of hypercortisolism, our endocrinological criteria for remission were either a suppression of cortisol levels to below 2 µg/dl or transient adrenocortical insufficiency due to a lack of ACTH secretion. According to these criteria, 13 out of our 14 patients had a remission following transsphenoidal adenomectomy of a microadenoma (Fig. 2).

In one patient no adenoma was found; in another adenomectomy failed to eliminate the ACTH excess. Both were submitted to bilateral adrenalectomy as soon as it was noted that transsphenoidal microsurgery had failed to eliminate hypercortisolism.

Follow-up of the patients ranged from 8 months to 7 years and was 3.7 years on an average. No recurrence was seen in the follow-up of patients operated on successfully. In all three girls with secondary amenorrhea menstruation recurred following pituitary microsurgery. Five out of the six patients with primary amenorrhea are having regular periods now. One of these patients—still amenorrhoic—was operated on recently. Catch-up growth or resumption of a normal growth rate was found in 8 of the 11 patients; all underwent selective adenomectomy before epiphyseal fusion had occurred.

The clinical remission of these symptoms due to restoration of impaired anterior pituitary function is prove of the selectivity of the surgical procedure. This

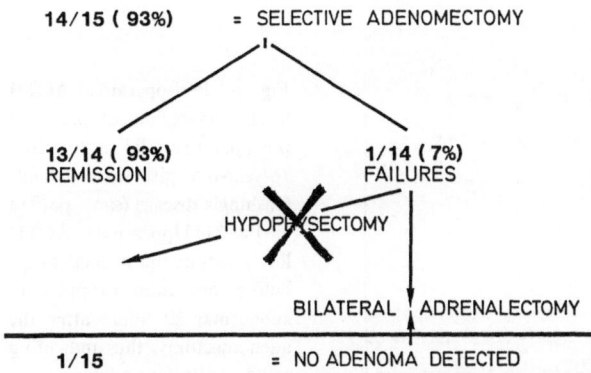

Fig. 2. 15 patients with Cushing's disease in childhood and adolescence: survey of the outcome of transsphenoidal surgery. In operative failures bilateral adrenalectomy is advocated instead of hypophysectomy

has also been demonstrated by dynamic endocrinological evaluation before and after surgery in all of the patients. Fig. 3 illustrates one example.

Peri-operative ACTH measurements[3] were done in all but one of the patients and proved to be very helpful in evaluating remission or failure and adrenocortical insufficiency. This occurred in all of the patients operated on successfully, but was never found to be permanent (Fig. 3). The response of ACTH secretion after administration of corticotropin releasing hormone gives additional information (Fig. 4).

Functional endocrinological testing showed that there was no deterioration of anterior pituitary function

except transient adrenocortical insufficiency, in general documenting a remission after the surgical procedure. Due to the low cortisol levels successfully operated patients required transient hydrocortisone replacement. Prophylactically corticosteroids are given to all patients just after the adenomectomy in order to prevent severe acute metabolic disturbances (e.g., hypoglycemia and hypotension).

Complications

Although most of the patients were regarded as high operative risks because of their reduced general resistance and metabolic dysregulations, we never refused surgery regardless of the severity of the disease. The death of a 16-year-old boy with a 9-year-history of Cushing's disease may be attributed to this fact. He was extremely overweight (102 kg) and had suffered from respiratory distress syndrome of 4 year's standing even prior to surgery. During the first week the postoperative course was uneventful. He died 4 weeks later of pneumonia resistant to antibiotics. Otherwise there was no serious morbidity, especially no CSF fistula, no meningitis, no phlebothrombosis and no pulmonary embolism.

Discussion

As neuroradiological evaluation of the sella turcica and the pituitary gland is still not a reliable method for

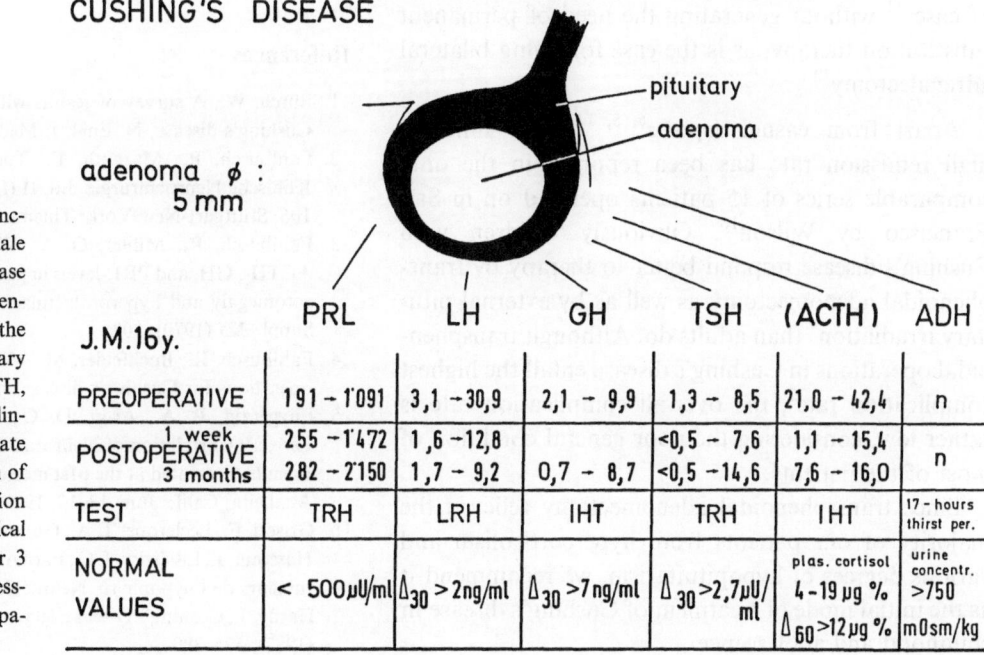

Fig. 3. Anterior pituitary function in a 16-year-old female with juvenile Cushing's disease before and after selective adenomectomy. The findings of the combined anterior pituitary stimulation test using ACTH, TRH, and LRH and insulin-induced hypoglycemia indicate that there is no deterioration of anterior pituitary function except transient adrenocortical insufficiency improving after 3 months and indicating a successful surgical procedure (same patient as Fig. 4)

SELECTIVE ADENOMECTOMY OF A MICROADENOMA IN CUSHING'S DISEASE

adenoma ϕ : 5 mm

J.M. 16 y.	PRL	LH	GH	TSH	(ACTH)	ADH
PREOPERATIVE	191 – 1'091	3,1 – 30,9	2,1 – 9,9	1,3 – 8,5	21,0 – 42,4	n
POSTOPERATIVE 1 week	255 – 1'472	1,6 – 12,8		<0,5 – 7,6	1,1 – 15,4	n
POSTOPERATIVE 3 months	282 – 2'150	1,7 – 9,2	0,7 – 8,7	<0,5 – 14,6	7,6 – 16,0	
TEST	TRH	LRH	IHT	TRH	IHT	17 – hours thirst per.
NORMAL VALUES	< 500 μU/ml	Δ_{30} >2ng/ml	Δ_{30} >7 ng/ml	Δ_{30} >2,7 μU/ml	plas. cortisol 4 – 19 μg % Δ_{60} >12 μg %	urine concentr. >750 mOsm/kg

Perioperative ACTH levels

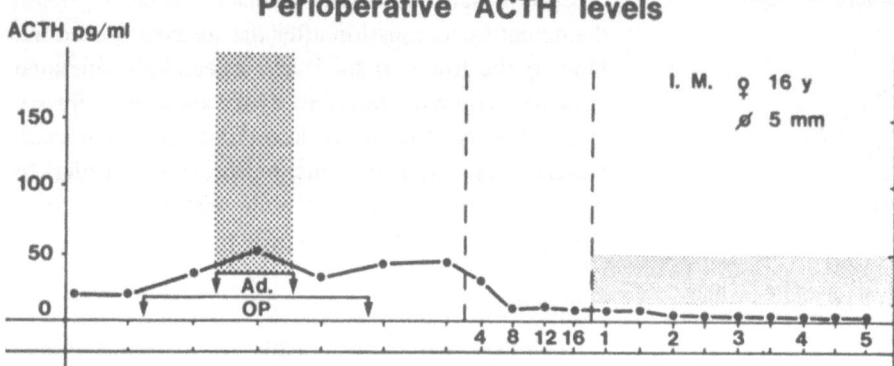

CRF - TEST

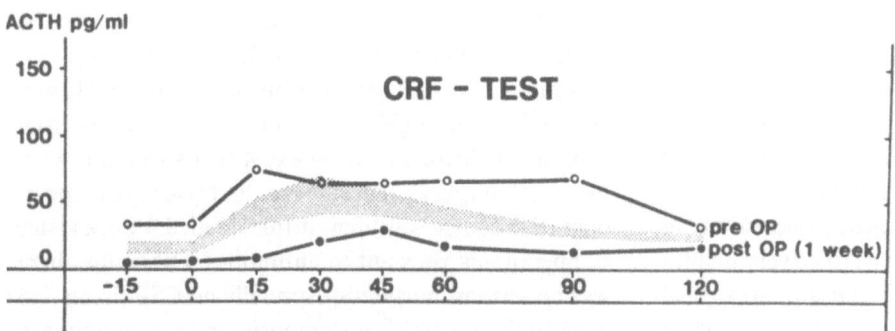

Fig. 4. Peri-operative ACTH levels and results of pre- and postoperative CRF testing in a 16-year-old girl with juvenile Cushing's disease (same patient as Fig. 3). Upper part: ACTH levels within the normal range before operation dropped to subnormal 20 hours after the adenomectomy, thus indicating acute pituitary-adrenal insufficiency. *Ad* adenomectomy; *OP* operation. Lower part: The response of ACTH following bolus injection of CRF is higher in comparison to normal individuals (dotted) before the operation but blunted one week post-operatively. Thus, pituitary-adrenocortical insufficiency indicates successful adenomectomy documented by CRF testing in this case. *pre OP* preoperatively; *post OP* postoperatively

confirming the presence of pituitary microadenoma in Cushing's disease[4, 5], the diagnosis of ACTH-secreting microadenomas is solely based on the results of dynamic endocrine testing[2, 12, 13]. The suppression of cortisol after low and high-dose dexamethasone still seems to be the most valuable test[13]. Apart from the remission of hypercortisolism restitution of anterior pituitary function can be achieved in a high percentage of cases[11] without generating the need of permanent substitution therapy, as is the case following bilateral adrenalectomy[10].

Apart from casual reports[6, 8, 14, 17] a similarly high remission rate has been reported in the only comparable series of 15 patients operated on in San Francisco by Wilson[16]. Obviously children with Cushing's disease respond better to therapy by transphenoidal adenomectomy as well as by external pituitary irradiation[9] than adults do. Although transphenoidal operations in Cushing's disease entail the highest complication rate[2], the over-all complication rate is rather low, considering the poor general condition of most of the patients.

Since transsphenoidal adenomectomy relieved the majority of our patients from hypercortisolism and various degrees of hypopituitarism, we recommend it as the initial mode of treatment of Cushing's disease in childhood and adolescence.

Acknowledgements

We are indebted to Prof. Dr. D. Knorr, Munich, Dr. W. Sippel, Kiel, and all other paediatricians and endocrinologists who made this work possible by referring their patients. We are also indebted to Dr. OA Müller and Dr. GK Stalla, Medizinische Klinik Innenstadt der Universität, Munich, and to Dr. U. Schrell, Neurochirurgische Klinik der Universität, Erlangen, for the determinations of ACTH levels in this series.

References

1. Burch, W., A survey of results with transphenoidal surgery in Cushing's disease, N. Engl. J. Med. *308* (1983), 103.
2. Fahlbusch, R., Marguth, F., Tumoren der Hypophyse. In: Klinische Neurochirurgie, Bd. II (Dietz H., *et al.,* eds.), pp. 86–106. Stuttgart-New York: Thieme. 1984.
3. Fahlbusch, R., Müller, O. A., Werder, K. v., Perioperative ACTH-, GH, and PRL-levels in patients with Cushing's disease, acromegaly and hyperprolactinaemia. Acta Endocrinol (Kbh) Suppl. *225* (1979), 202.
4. Fahlbusch, R., Buchfelder, M., Müller, O.A., Transsphenoidal operations for Cushing's disease, J. Roy. Soc. Med., in press.
5. Fitzgerald, P. A., Aron, D. C., Findling, J. W., Cushing's Disease: Correlation of Neuroradiological Studies and Surgical Results. Presented at the 61st meeting of the Endocrine Society, Anaheim, Calif., June 13–15, 1979.
6. Grisoli, F., Leclerque, T. A., Guibout, M., Jaquet, P., Heim, M., Hassoun, J., Lissitzky, J. C., Farnarier, P., Maladie de Cushing et tumeurs de l'hypophyse. Neurochirurgie *25* (1979) 3–10.
7. Hardy, J., Cushing's Disease: 50 years later. Can. J. Neurol. Sci. *9* (1982), 375–380.

8. Houwen, R. H. J., Drop, S. L. S., Hazebroek, F. W. J., Ten Kate, F. W. J., Pituitary-dependent Cushing's disease and primary adrenocortical nodular dysplasia in childhood. Eur. J. Paediatr. *141* (1983) 101–108.

9. Jennings, A. S., Liddle, G. W., Orth, A. N., Results of treating childhood Cushing's disease with pituitary irradiation, N. Engl. J. Med. *297* (1977), 957–962.

10. Kelly, W. F., McFarlane, J. A., Longson, D., Davies, D., Sutcliffe, H., Cushing's disease treated by total adrenalectomy: long-term observations of 43 patients., Q. J. Med. *206* (1983), 224–231.

11. Kuwayama, A., Kageyama, N., Nakane, T., Watanabe, M., Kanie, N., Anterior pituitary function after transsphenoidal selective adenomectomy in patients with Cushing's disease. J. Clin. Endocrinol. Metabol. *53* (1981), 165–173.

12. Müller, O. A., Fahlbusch, R., Zur Diagnose und Therapie des hypothalamo-hypophysären Cushing-Syndroms—derzeitiger Stand und neue Aspekte. Acta Endocrinol. Stoffw. *5* (1984), 142–147.

13. Liddle, G. W., Tests of pituitary-adrenal suppressibility in the diagnosis of Cushing's syndrome. J. Clin. Endocrinol. Metabol. *20* (1960), 1539–1560.

14. Nolan, P. N., Sheeler, L. R., Hahn, J. F., Hardy, R. W., Therapeutic problems with transphenoidal pituitary surgery for Cushing's disease. Cleveland Clin. Quart. *49* (1982), 199–207.

15. Sippel, W., Kinet, M., Pfeiffer, J., Knorr, D., Fahlbusch, R., Therapie des zentralen Morbus Cushing im Kindesalter durch transsphenoidale Resektion hypophysärer Mikroadenome, 77. Tagung der Dt. Ges. Kinderheilkunde, Düsseldorf 1981. (Abstract.)

16. Styne, D. M., Grumbach, M. M., Kaplan, S. L., Wilson, C. B., Conte, F. A., Treatment of Cushing's disease in childhood and adolescence by transsphenoidal microsurgery, N. Engl. J. Med. *310* (1984), 889–893.

17. Werder, E. A., Girard, J., Zachmann, M., Illig, R., Landolt, A. M., Treatment of Cushing's disease in childhood by resection of a pituitary microadenoma. International Symposium on Pituitary Microadenomas, Milano, 1978. (Abstract.)

Author's address: Dr. Michael Buchfelder, Neurochirurgische Klinik der Universität Erlangen-Nürnberg, Schwabachanlage 6, D-8520 Erlangen, Federal Republic of Germany.

Acta Neurochirurgica, Suppl. 35, 106–110 (1985)

Gliomas of Visual Pathways and Hypothalamus in Children— A Preliminary Report

F. Helcl[1] and H. Petrásková[2]

[1] Department of Paediatric Neurosurgery, Paediatric Teaching Hospital, Prague, ČSSR
[2] The Neurological Clinic, CT Department, Faculty Hospital, Prague, ČSSR

Summary

26 children with gliomas of the visual pathway and hypothalamus were seen during 5 years. 4 of them had intraorbital tumors, in 22 children tumors were localized in the chiasmal/hypothalamic regions. In 25 patients the tumors were surgically explored. All 4 intraorbital gliomas were radically removed using a transcranial approach. Exploration without biopsy was performed 7 times, exploration plus limited biopsy in 3 cases. In the remaining 11 operated children partial or subtotal removal of the tumor was possible. One of the 18 histologically verified tumors was an anaplastic glioma, the others were typical pilocytic astrocytomas. 12 children had hydrocephalus. 7 patients died, 19 are still alive. The operative mortality was 4 out of our 25 operated cases (16%). All of these patients had large tumors with posterior spread into the hypothalamus. In future, surgery in these children should be confined to exploration and limited biopsy followed by radiotherapy. We advocate exploration and biopsy in all chiasmal/hypothalamic tumors. The growth potential of these tumors is individually variable. We recommend to follow-up all patients at 3 months' intervals by means of visual evoked potentials, visual acuity, fundoscopy and visual field testing. CT scans and X-rays of the optic canals should be performed once a year. Surgery should only be considered if clinical and/or neuroradiological progression has been documented.

Keywords: Optic nerve glioma; chiasmal/hypothalamic region; extent of surgery; follow-up methods.

Gliomas of the visual pathways and hypothalamus have been a controversial issue for neurosurgeons for decades. Many have advocated radical surgery (Housepian[2]); others consider surgery to be indicated (Till[16], Koos[6], Northfield[11]); the approach of Hoyt and Baghdassarian[3]) is extremely conservative; some authors have reported beneficial effects of irradiation (Taveras[14]). We saw a series of 26 children in a relatively short period of 5 years. This unusual concentration prompted us to analyze these cases and present our experience, especially those with surgery. The purpose of this report is to review our surgical indications in correlation with CT findings, extent of surgery, total and operative mortality and its causes. Clinical signs and symptoms, oncologic therapy and management of hydrocephalus are summarized in Tables. Finally our follow-up methods and their schedule are described. As our follow-up period is relatively short (from 2 months to 6 years and 9 months) detailed ophthalmological results are not reliable enough for inclusion in this report.

Methods and Materials

26 children were admitted to the Department of Neurosurgery, Paediatric Teaching Hospital, Prague 5, Motol, between 1st January, 1979 and 30th September, 1984 with the diagnosis of glioma of the visual pathways and hypothalamus. This series includes all patients with tumors localized in one optic nerve (either intraorbitally or intracranially) and tumors arising from the chiasm and/or hypothalamus with extension into the visual pathways. Children with glial tumors in the region of the third ventricle not invading the visual pathways were excluded.

The medical records, operation protocols, death certificates and outpatient records of these 26 patients were reviewed. CT scans were reexamined by one of us (H. P.). All available oncologic data were collected from the departments where patients were irradiated.

The operative approach was transcranial in all cases (Dandy[1], Kempe[5], Housepian[2]). All intraorbital tumors were totally removed after removing the orbital roof. In addition to total mortality, operative mortality was computed. It was defined as deaths causally related to the surgical procedure within 1 day to 2 months after surgery. Tumor size and posterior spread into the hypothalamus were correlated with the post-operative course and the extent of surgery.

Results

Out of our 26 patients with gliomas of the visual pathways and hypothalamus, 4 had tumors involving only one optic nerve and 22 had chiasmal and/or hypothalamic involvement. This series contained 15 males (57.7%) and 11 females (42.3%). The age ranged from 4 months to 13.5 years, mean age was 5 years and 4 months. Presenting symptoms are summarized in Table 1. They included poor vision (8), squint (4), hypothalamic dystrophy (4), intracranial hypertension (3), nystagmus (2), proptosis (2), behavioural changes (2) and vertigo (1).

Table 1. *Clinical Signs and Symptoms*

Poor vision	8
Squint	4
Hypothalamic dystrophy	4
Intracranial hypertension	3
Nystagmus	2
Proptosis	2
Behavioral changes	2
Vertigo	1
Total	26

All 4 patients with *intraorbital gliomas of the optic nerve* were operated on by a transcranial approach after removing the roof of the orbit (Dandy[1]). The average duration of the history was 5.4 months in this group, the age ranged from 6 months to 13 years and 7 months, the mean age was 6 years and 10 months. All of these patients were alive at the time of this report. None had signs of progression of the tumor into the chiasm or into the opposite optic nerve (Figs. 1 and 2).

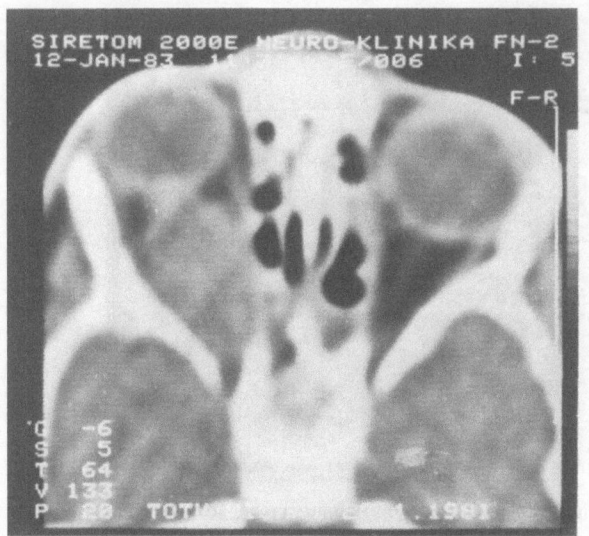

Fig. 1. Axial CT scan showing intraorbital left optic nerve glioma

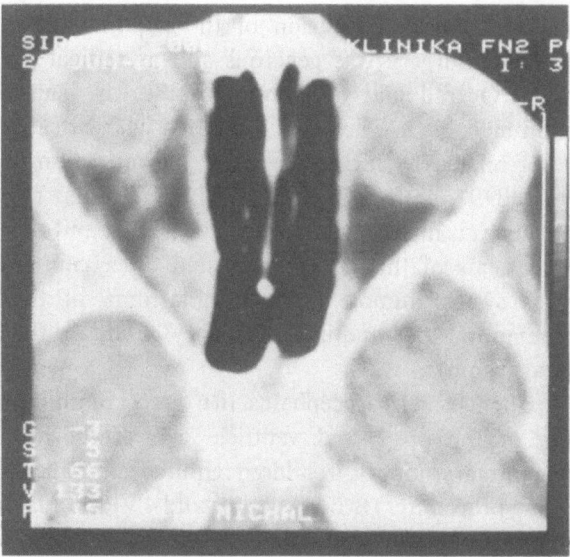

Fig. 2. Axial CT scan of patient in Fig. 1 after total removal of the tumor transcranially. Note hyperdensity of extraocular muscles in the apex of left orbit. Distinguishing it from tumor recurrence is very difficult

There were 22 children in the group of *chiasmal and/or hypothalamic tumors*. Their age ranged from 4 months to 12 years and 5 months (mean 5 years and 1 month). The average duration of the history was 10 months. 21 patients of this group were operated on. In 11 children we performed subtotal or partial removal of their tumors, in 3 others the chiasmal region was explored and a small tumor fragment was removed for evaluation. In 7 cases exploratory craniotomy was performed for revision of the chiasm without taking a biopsy. One patient was not operated on at all, but underwent radiotherapy. 7 patients died. In 4 of them death was causally related to surgery (operative mortality, 16%). Modalities of surgical treatment are listed in Table 2.

Table 2. *Modalities of Surgical Treatment*

Total removal (unilateral optic nerve glioma)	4
Subtotal or partial removal	11
Exploration of chiasm and biopsy	3
Exploration of chiasm without biopsy	7
No operation on tumor	1
Total	26

The operative mortality was relatively high (16%) and needs more detailed explanation. All of these 4 non surviving children had large tumors in the chiasmal region with marked invasion of the hypothalamus posteriorly. Surgery was generous and as radical as possible. Overall and operative mortality are summarized in Table 3. The other 3 children whose death was not related to surgery survived the operation 4 years and 9 months, 2 years and 5.5 months, respectively. It is interesting to note that the first and the third patients of this latter group had other central nervous system tumors (ependymoblastoma of the right temporal lobe and intramedullary glioma in the cervical region).

12 patients had hydrocephalus. In 6 direct communication of the obstructed ventricle was established during primary surgery, 6 children required subsequent shunting procedures (two VA shunts and 4 VP shunts); the management of hydrocephalus is shown in Table 4.

Table 3. *Operative Mortality*

Name	Death after operation
1. Z. P.	2 months
2. P. H.	12 days
3. M. S.	12 hours
4. P. H.	24 hours
Total	4 out of 25 surgical cases (16%)

Survival of 3 patients who died later

5. P. M.	4 years and 9 months
6. O. H.	2 years
7. M. S.	5.5 months

Table 4. *Surgery of Hydrocephalus*

Direct communication of obstructed ventricle	6
VA shunt	2
VP shunt	4
Total	12

18 patients with tumors in the chiasmal and/or hypothalamic regions were irradiated, 6 of them also underwent repeated courses of chemotherapy. In 8 patients irradiation of the tumor was the only therapy. Oncologic therapy is briefly summarized in Table 5. Detailed results will be published elsewhere.

Table 5. *Oncologic Therapy*

Irradiation only	12
Irradiation plus chemotherapy	6
No oncology therapy	8
Total cases	26
Oncologic therapy alone (tumor not operated)	8

Discussion

Gliomas of the visual pathways and hypothalamus have been a major therapeutic problem for neurosurgeons, radiotherapists and ophthalmic surgeons for many decades. In some reports an active surgical approach was recommended (Housepian[2], Till[16], Koos[6], Northfield[11]). This policy has changed in 1969 after Hoyt's and Baghdassarian's papers advocating conservative management. These authors reserved surgery for the treatment of hydrocephalus and the relief of severe proptosis of a blind eye. They even rejected exploratory craniotomies (before the advent of CT) as well as radiotherapy. Our approach, *i.e.,* to explore all tumors, is the same as that of Northfield[11]. He stated that "a small filling defect in the third ventricle should not necessarily be interpreted as an inoperable extension into the chiasm, because the intracranial portion of an optic nerve glioma may compress and displace the chiasm without invading it". We fully agree with this statement and Figs. 3 and 4 demonstrate the successful

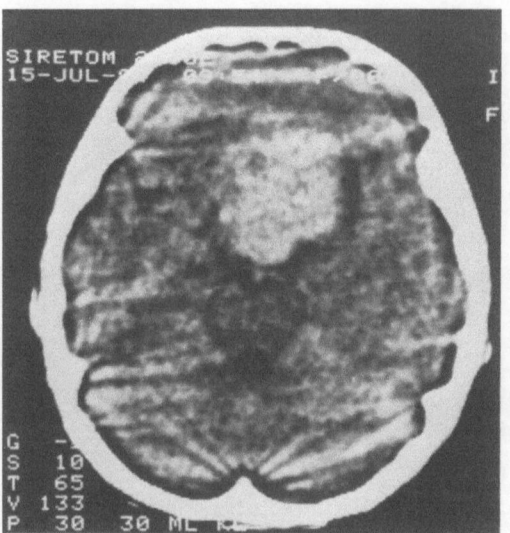

Fig. 3. Axial CT scan of huge tumor arising from the right optic nerve and right half of the chiasm and compressing left optic nerve. Note positive enhancement

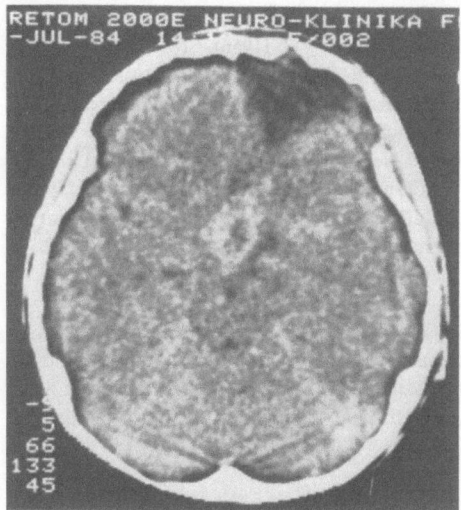

Fig. 4. Axial CT scan of the patient in Fig. 3 after subtotal removal of the tumor, small part of it was left behind in the chiasm

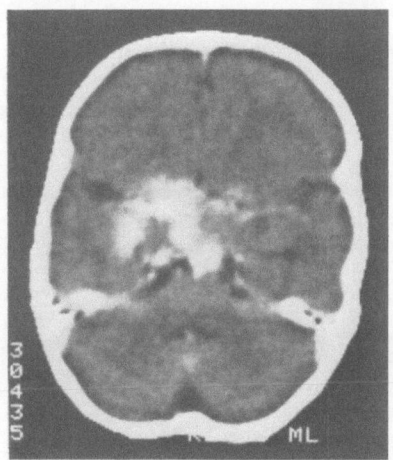

Fig. 5. Axial CT scan of the patient who died 12 hours after radical surgery. Note extent of tumor in chiasmal region and marked posterior spread into hypothalamus

We support Wrights[17] conclusion that the natural history of these tumors is not necessarily stable. In some cases progressive deterioration of visual functions may be present. In these, an active approach, either surgical or radiotherapeutical, is justified. In the "stable" group it is advisable to wait for some time and evaluate the individual growth potential of the tumor, before deciding for surgery and/or radiotherapy. This policy is especially important in children with unilateral optic nerve gliomas if vision of the affected eye is still good and proptosis minimal. The same conclusion was drawn by Tenny[15] from the Mayo Clinic. We recommend to examine visual acuity, visual field, optic discs and visual evoked potentials (VEP) every 3 months in these patients. CT scans and X-rays of the optic canals should be repeated at least once a year unless clinical deterioration requires shorter intervals. Our experience with irradiation of inoperable tumors is promising, but beyond the scope of this report. In small children we have used a more active surgical approach and will continue to do so, because testing of visual function and/or VEP is not reliable enough. This has also been advocated by Oxenhandler and Sayers[12]. An individualized approach in each and every patient is inevitable as has been emphasized by these authors.

Acknowledgement

The authors are grateful to Dr. Stejskal and Dr. Julisova from the Department of Pathology, Paediatric Faculty in Prague, for reviewing all histological specimens.

We appreciate the kind help of Dr. Koutecky from the Paediatric Oncology Clinic, Paediatric Teaching Hospital, Prague 5, Motol, in oncologic questions.

subtotal removal of a huge tumor in the chiasmal region arising from the right optic nerve and the right half of the chiasm and compressing the left optic nerve.

The presence of anaplastic glioma, which is extremely rare in children, has prompted us to take a small particle of tumor tissue for biopsy in all future patients undergoing exploratory surgery.

Our operative mortality is relatively high (16%). The relevant patients had large chiasmal tumors with marked posterior extension into the hypothalamus. In such cases extensive surgery is not advisable. In future, we will explore all of these lesions, but we will only perform limited biopsies. An example of such a tumor is shown in Fig. 5.

References

1. Dandy, W. E., Surgery of the Brain, pp. 650–667. Hagerstown, Maryland: W.F. Prior Comp. Inc. 1945.
2. Housepian, E. M., Surgical treatment of unilateral optic nerve gliomas. J. Neurosurg. 31 (1969), 604–607.
3. Hoyt, W. F., Baghdassarian, S. A., Optic nerve glioma of childhood: natural history and rationale for conservative management. Brit. J. Ophthal. 53 (1969), 793–798.
4. Ingraham, F. D., Matson, D. D., Neurosurgery of Infancy and Childhood, pp. 331–342. Springfield, Ill.: Ch. C Thomas 1954.
5. Kempe, L. G., Operative Neurosurgery, Vol. 1, pp. 76–78. Berlin-Heidelberg-New York: Springer. 1968.
6. Koos, W. Th., Böck, F. W., Spetzler, R. F., Clinical Microneurosurgery, pp. 58–63. Stuttgart: Thieme. 1976.
7. Kunc, Z., Neurochirurgie, 3rd ed., pp. 142. Praha: Avicenum. 1983.

8. McCarty, C. S., Boyd, A. S., Childs, D. S., Tumors of the optic nerve and optic chiasm. J. Neurosurg. *33* (1970), 439–444.

9. McDonnell, P., Miller, H. R., Chiasmatic and hypothalamic extension of optic nerve glioma. Arch. Ophthalmol. *101* (1983), 1412–1415.

10. Miller, N. R., Iliff, W. J., Green, W. R., Evaluation and management of gliomas of the anterior visual pathways. Brain *97* (1974), 743–754.

11. Northfield, D. W. C., The Surgery of the Central Nervous System, pp. 183–185. Oxford-London-Edinburgh-Melbourne: Blackwell Scientific Publ. 1973.

12. Oxenhandler, D. C., Sayers, M. P., The dilemma of childhood optic glioma. J. Neurosurg. *48* (1978), 34–41.

13. Rush, J. A., Younge, B. R., Campbell, R. J., Optic glioma: long-term follow up of 85 histopathologically verified cases. Ophthalmology *89* (1982), 1213–1219.

14. Taveras, J. M., Mount, L. A., Wood, E. H., The value of radiation therapy in the management of glioma of the optic nerves and chiasm. Radiology *66* (1956), 518–528.

15. Tenny, R. T., Laws, E. R., jr., Younge, B. R., Rush, J. A., The neurosurgical management of optic glioma. J. Neurosurg. *57* (1982), 452–458.

16. Till, K., Paediatric Neurosurgery, pp. 38–43. Oxford-London-Edinburgh-Melbourne: Blackwell Scientific Publ. 1975.

17. Wright, J. E., McDonald, W. I., Call, N. B., Management of optic nerve gliomas, Br. J. Ophthalmol. *64* (1980), 545–552.

Author's addresses: Dr. F. Helcl, Department of Paediatric Neurosurgery, Paediatric Teaching Hospital, V Úvalu 84, 150 18 Prague 5, Motol, ČSSR. Dr. H. Petrásková, The Neurological Clinic, CT Depart., Faculty Hospital, Kateřinská 30, 120 00 Prague 2, ČSSR.

Acta Neurochirurgica, Suppl. 35, 111–113 (1985)

H. Pineal Region

Surgical Aspects of Pineal Region Tumors in Children

G. Broere

Department of Neurosurgery, Academic Hospital of the Vrije Universiteit, Amsterdam, The Netherlands

Summary

The use of the operating microscope and specialized anesthesiologic techniques make it possible to operate safely on tumors in the pineal region. A survey is presented of the main surgical and anesthesiologic techniques used: the supracerebellar infratentorial approach in the sitting position and the occipital transtentorial approach in the semi-sitting position. For selecting the optimal approach a CT scan with sagittal sections is very important to localize the tumor in relation to the tentorium cerebelli, the straight sinus and the great vein of Galen. Based upon the comparison of the two techniques the author concludes that nearly all tumors in the pineal region in children can be operated by the infratentorial supracerebellar route and that the transtentorial route offers relatively little advantage.

Keywords: Tumors of the pineal region; operative approaches; infratentorial versus transtentorial.

Introduction and Historical Review

In the last fifteen years the operative aspects of tumors in the pineal region have been extensively discussed and several publications can be found on this subject. Till 1975 most authors faced with tumors associated with hydrocephalus opted for ventricular drainage followed by radiotherapy.

The increasing use of the operating microscope and improvements in neuroanesthesiology revived interest in the infratentorial supracerebellar approach as originally described by Krause in 1926 and in the occipital transtentorial route published by Heppner[3] in 1959 and Poppen[7] in 1960. In the following years these two techniques were extended: In 1971 Stein[11] used the infratentorial supracerebellar approach for pineal lesions in 6 children from 8 months to 14 years. As a result of his positive experience with it he recommended that all pineal tumors should be explored prior to considering radiotherapy.

The transtentorial occipital route was refined by Glasauer[2] in 1970. He fashioned an osteoplastic bone flap attached to the occipital muscles with the patient sitting. The boneflap crossed the midline 3 cm to the left and the left lateral ventricle was drained. It is essential to retract the occipital lobe laterally and upward, thus exposing the angle between the posterior falx and the medial part of the tentorium, which is opened parallel to the straight sinus. With this technique it is possible to open the dura on both sides of the falx. But as bilateral exploration appeared to be of no benefit, it has no longer been considered necessary in later publications.

In 1974 Lazar and Kemp Clark[5] recommended right occipital craniotomy to just over the superior sagittal and the right transverse sinuses. They operated on the patient in the sitting position.

In Europe and America pinealomas account for no more than 0.4–0.7% of all cerebral tumors. Therefore, it is difficult to gather extensive experience with the operative approaches to these tumors.

The microsurgical anatomy encountered on microsurgical dissection was described by Quest and Kleriga[8] in 1980.

Should preference be given to one of these techniques if you have both at your disposal?

In 1978 Reid and Kemp Clark[9] compared the 2 techniques in 15 patients with the infratentorial supracerebellar route used in 4 and the occipital transtentorial approach in 11 of them. Their series was mainly composed of adults. Because of the sometimes limited space in the tentorial hiatus they decided in favor of the occipital transtentorial approach in the sitting position, although the resultant lesions of the occipital lobe caused visual field defects in 2 of their 11 patients.

Page[6] in 1977 found the infratentorial exposure excellent for lesions in the pineal region because it was less hampered by the vein of Galen and its tributaries than the transtentorial operation. But lesions extending above the tentorium cannot be reached by this method. Sano[10] (1981) mainly used the transtentorial approach on the non-dominant side in the prone position, since this provided access for both low and high parieto-occipital exploration along the midline and left the infratentorial route for small tumors.

In 1984 Barba and James[1] recommended the occipital transtentorial approach in pediatric patients for tumors of the anterior part of the fourth ventricle and cerebellum. In this paper a comparison is made between the infratentorial and transtentorial exposures.

Material and Methods

Between January 1978 and June 1984 6 pediatric patients underwent surgery by the infratentorial supracerebellar approach. One of them had received radiotherapy one year before the operation for a suspected tumor in the pineal region, which had not been verified histologically. In three children the transtentorial route was used. The age of the children ranged from 4 to 14 years. Ventriculoperitoneal drainage was instituted throughout prior to the exploration of the tumor because of obstructive hydrocephalus.

The symptoms of tumors in the pineal region included signs of increased intracranial pressure, signs of encroachment on neighbouring parts of the brain, disturbances of growth and development (in less than 10%).

The diagnosis was based upon clinical, laboratory and neuroradiologic investigations. Assaying for the tumor markers alphafetoprotein (AFP) and human gonadotropin (HCG) was thought to be essential.

Neuroradiology consisted of a CT scan before and after ventriculoperitoneal shunting. The postprocedural CT should include horizontal and coronal as well as sagittal scans. In the saggital slices the relation of the tumor to the tentorial hiatus, the great vein of Galen, the third and fourth ventricles, the brain stem and cerebellar vermis is distinctly seen. This is important for the route of access. The information acquired by CT is better than that provided by late venous phase cerebral angiography.

To reduce the risk of cerebral edema during the operation Oradexon (dexamethason) was started the evening before surgery (2.5–5 mg), continued at a dose of 2.5 mg t.i.d. for the next three days and then tapered. At the beginning of the operation mannitole 0.5 g/kg bodyweight, was administered.

The position of the patient on the operating table is important (see Table 1).

Most operating tables are not suited for pediatric patients. A vaccum cushion can help to solve this problem. It supports the patient very well in this difficult position.

Iodine ointment was used to seal the headpins and surroundings of the Mayfield headrest in order to prevent potential air embolism along the headpin to a diploic skull vein.

Table 1. *Position of the Patient on the Operating Table*

Supracerebellar infratentorial	Occipital transtentorial
Sitting	Semi-sitting
Orbito-inion line: 30 degrees	Orbito-inion line: horizontal
Mayfield headrest	Mayfield headrest
Vacuum cushion	Vacuum cushion
Legs wrapped	Legs wrapped
Microscope: objective 250/300 mm	Microscope: objective 300 mm

Table 2. *Anesthesiologic Monitoring Program During Pineal Tumor Surgery in the Sitting or Semi-Sitting Positions*

Positive end-expiratory pressure (PEEP)
Pulse and ECG
Arterial pressure
Central venous pressure
Capnography
Doppler
Temperature
If indicated: Swan-Ganz catheter for hemodynamic monitoring

Table 3. *Post-operative Checks After Operations in the Pineal Region*

Consciousness; E.M.V. scale
Arterial pressure
Pulse and ECG
Temperature
Bloodgas analysis
If indicated: intracranial pressure

The anesthesiologic parameters are summarized in Table 2.

As we never saw any serious air embolism during operations on pediatric patients in a sitting or semi-sitting position, we cannot comment on the effectiveness of aspirating air by way of the central venous line or the Swan-Ganz catheter.

All operations were performed as described by Stein[11] and by Lazar and Kemp Clark[5].

The post-operative checks are listed in Table 3.

As all our patients had a functioning ventriculoperitoneal shunt at the time of surgery we did not check the intracranial pressure.

Results

There was no mortality. Patients were mobilized within 3 days of the operation. Oculomotor disorders improved, but did not entirely disappear. One of the three patients undergoing transtentorial surgery developed a transient visual defect attributable to the lesions in the right occipital lobe.

In the child with prior radiotherapy no further treatment was scheduled for what was a teratoma histologically. The histologic diagnosis in the other cases was: pinealoma (7) and germinoma (1).

Post-operative CT showed residual tumor tissue in 4 of the infratentorial and all three of the transtentorial cases. The two children without residual tumors by CT were seen in the early period when CT images were less distinct, but what we saw at surgery supported that a small residual tumor mass had been left attached to the brain-stem. All patients without previous radiotherapy were scheduled for post-operative irradiation.

Discussion

Accurate pre-operative localization of the tumor with respect to the surrounding structures is imperative. Sagittal reconstruction of the horizontal and coronal CT scans is not clear enough. Direct sagittal scans give more conclusive information and are readily obtained in co-operative and mobile children.

In all our patients tumor localization would have been compatible with both the infratentorial supracerebellar and the transtentorial occipital approaches. The frontal transcallosal approach described by Sano[10] for huge tumors was ruled out in our material.

Based upon earlier experiences with the infratentorial route in adults, we first considered this approach to be superior to the transtentorial access, but later found the transtentorial route to be equally useful.

Although we were extremely careful while working our way along the occipital lobe during the transtentorial operation, the lobe was still injured in one of our patients. The result was a visual field defect in terms of left hemianopia, which disappeared almost completely within three months.

The advantages and disadvantages of the two operative techniques are summarized in Table 4.

Bases on the experiences in the literature and on our own observations, we conclude that nearly all tumors in the pineal region can be operated safely along the infratentorial supracerebellar route. The transtentorial route offers little advantage.

Both operative techniques are time-consuming and demanding for both the patient and the operating team. Subsequent radiotherapy is often necessary.

The merits of such recent developments as CT-guided systems should be weighed against open surgery for making a histologic diagnosis. However, both operative techniques will also be of value for the

Table 4

Supracerebellar infratentorial approach; sitting patient	Occipital transtentorial approach; semi-sitting patient
	versus

Advantages	
Nearly atraumatic access; good view of midline struct.; low intravenous pressure;	Operative field is 1 cm less deep than infratentorial; low intravenous pressure; extension to paramedian transcallosal route possible

Disadvantages	
Poor view of large tumors with basal extension; risk of air embolism surgeons's position tiring	Risk of occipital lobe injury orientation sometimes difficult; narrow access when basal veins are pushed up; risk of air embolism

exploration of tumors in patients who are not candidates for radiotherapy.

References

1. Barba, D., James, H. E., The occipital transtentorial approach to the posterior fossa in the paediatric patient. Childs Brain *11* (1984), 145–154.
2. Glassauer, F. E., An operative approach to pineal tumors. Acta Neurochir. (Wien) *22* (1970), 177–180.
3. Heppner, F., Zur Operationstechnik bei Pinaleomen. Zbl. Neurochir. *19* (1959), 219–224.
4. Krause, F., Operative Freilegung der Vierhügel, nebst Beobachtungen über Hirndruck und Decompression. Zentralbl. Chir. *53* (1926), 2812–2819.
5. Lazar, M. L., Kemp Clark, W., Direct surgical management of masses in the region of the vein of Galen. Surg. Neurol. *2* (1974), 17–21.
6. Page, L. K., The infratentorial supracerebellar exposure of tumors in the pineal area. Neurosurgery *1* (1977), 36–40.
7. Poppen, J. L., An Atlas of Neurosurgical Techniques, 130–133. Philadelphia: W. B. Saunders. 1960.
8. Quest, D. O., Kleriga, E., Microsurgical anatomy of the pineal region. Neurosurgery *6* (1980), 385–390.
9. Reid, W. S., Kemp Clark, W., Comparison of the infratentorial and transtentorial approaches to the pineal region. Neurosurgery *3* (1978), 1–8.
10. Sano, K., Matsutani, M., Pinealoma (germinoma) treated by direct surgery and post-operative irradiation. Childs Brain *8* (1981), 81–97.
11. Stein, B. M., The infratentorial supracerebellar approach to pineal lesions. J. Neurosurg. *35* (1971), 197–202.

Author's address: Dr. G. Broere, Akademisch Ziekenhuis der Vrije Universiteit, de Boelelaan 1117, 1007 MB Amsterdam, The Netherlands.

Acta Neurochirurgica, Suppl. 35, 114–118 (1985)

Surgery of Pineal Region Lesions in Childhood

G. Pendl and **P. Vorkapic**

Department of Neurosurgery, University of Vienna Medical School, Wien, Austria

Summary

Personal experience with surgical exploration and total resection or evacuation of pineal and midbrain mass lesions in 20 pediatric patients from a total material of 52 cases demonstrate the efficacy of modern microsurgical techniques. Microtopography indicated the choice of the most suitable approach to these deep-seated lesions. The infratentorial supracerebellar approach proved to be the ideal exposure, except in one case of a lesion in the interpeduncular cistern, where a subtemporal approach was chosen. There was only one death as a consequence of the operation in a case of an extensive medulloblastoma; in all the other cases, no increase in morbidity occurred after surgery. Duration of post-operative observation with individual survival times will be demonstrated.

Keywords: Pediatric brain tumors; pineal region; midbrain region; microsurgery.

Introduction

Rational therapy in deep-seated lesions of the brain is only possible if the histology is known. Since these lesions are considered inoperable, they are often subjected to radiotherapy. Only in a few centers at least stereotactic biopsy is performed, but recent results on the reliability of mandatory smear preparations will promote this method in the future (Ostertag *et al.* 1980). Advanced techniques in microneurosurgery as well as in anesthesiology and intensive care have enabled neurosurgery to approach lesions of the midline with the aid of modern neuroimaging methods with gratifying results. Especially, lesions of the pineal region can now be safely attacked on the basis of a better understanding of microsurgical anatomy which was provided for greater safety. Since lesions arising from the posterior third ventricle and midbrain constitute a similar surgical challenge and often cannot be separated clinically and morphologically from "true" pineal tumors, they should be included in a study of pineal region lesions (Wood *et al.* 1981; Pendl 1985).

Material

Between 1973 and 1984 a total of 52 personal cases of pineal and midbrain lesions was seen and treated by the senior author (G. P.). 25 of them belonged to the pediatric age group and are the subject of this study. Table 1 lists lesions verified by open surgery and confined to the pineal region, *i.e.*, true classical pineal tumors, which accounted for 9 cases. Table 2 lists 11 lesions intrinsic to the midbrain and also verified by a direct surgical approach (Fig. 1). In 5 cases surgery was either refused or the lesions appeared to be inoperable by their clinical course and location (Table 3). The histological variety is shown in Table 4.

Method of Management

It is mandatory to select a uniform approach in the management of pineal region lesions. The traditional approach to this pathology by diversionary CSF shunt and radiotherapy is not used by the authors. Also, stereotactic biopsy has so far not been introduced, as the validity of this method for exact histological verification has not been convincing when compared to safe open exploration with modern neurosurgical equipment. Therefore, direct surgical approach by microsurgical techniques has been the treatment of choice of the senior author since 1973. In occlusive hydrocephalus, which was present in only 3 out of 9 pineal lesions and in 7 out of 11 cases with midbrain lesions VA shunt was only necessary once after surgery. The mode of surgical approach was infratentorial in all midbrain lesions except in a hamartoma of the interpeduncular cistern, where a subtemporal approach was used. In pineal masses an infratentorial supracerebellar approach was also employed except in two cases of large cystic lesions in infants, where transventricular fenestration seemed to be safer and less mutilating.

Operative death occured in one case with medulloblastoma extending from the vermis through the midbrain well into the third ventricle 2 months post-

Table 1. *Clinical Data in 9 Children With Direct Surgical Approach to Pineal Lesions*

Case no.	Age	Sex	Histology	Surgical approach	Additional therapy	Follow-up
1	8 months	m	medulloblastoma	infratentorial	radiotherapy chemotherapy	death from disease 2 years and 2 months
2	10 years	m	germinoma	infratentorial	radiotherapy	alive and well 4 years and 6 months
3	12 years	m	germinoma	infratentorial	radiotherapy	alive and well 3 years and 6 months
4	12 years	f	pineocytoma	infratentorial	none	alive and well 3 years
5	1 year 9 months	f	arachnoid cyst	transventricular	VA shunt	alive and well 2 years and 5 months
6	1 year	m	glial cyst	transventricular	VA shunt	alive and well 2 years
7	3 months	m	primitive neuro-ectodermal tumor	infratentorial	radiotherapy chemotherapy	death from disease 4 months
8	15 years	m	glial cyst	infratentorial	none	alive and well 1 year and 6 months
9	1 year 6 months	f	pilocytic astrocytoma	infratentorial	VA shunt	alive and well 15 months

Table 2. *Clinical Data in 11 Children With Direct Surgical Approach to Lesions Within the Midbrain*

Case no.	Age	Sex	Histology	Localization	Additional therapy	Follow-up
1	11 years	f	pilocytic astrocytoma	left cerebral peduncle	pre-operative radio-therapy, VA shunt	alive and well 11 years
2	9 years	m	ependymoblastoma	midbrain and poste-rior 3rd ventricle	pre-operative radio-therapy, Torkildsen	18 months death from disease
3	3 years	f	medulloblastoma	midbrain and poste-rior 3rd ventricle	post-operative radio-therapy, VA shunt	15 months death from disease
4	16 years	m	hamartoma	interpeduncular cistern	none	alive w. deficit 6 years
5	2 years	m	medulloblastoma	vermis—midbrain—post. 3rd ventricle	pre-operative VA shunt	death 2 months post-operative
6	5 years	m	astrocytoma II	4th ventricle and midbrain	post-operative radio-therapy	alive w. deficit 3 years
7	17 months	m	ependymoma I	4th ventricle and left midbrain	post-operative radio-therapy, VA shunt	alive and well 18 months
8	14 years	f	hematoma	right midbrain	pre-operative VA shunt	alive and well 18 months
9	16 years	m	pilocytic astrocytoma	midbrain	partial resection 6 years earlier with VA shunt	alive w. deficit 6 months
10	13 years	m	glial tumor	quadrigeminal plate	pre-operative VA shunt	alive and well 3 months
11	5 years	m	astrocytoma III	left midbrain	post-operative radio-therapy	alive and well 1 month

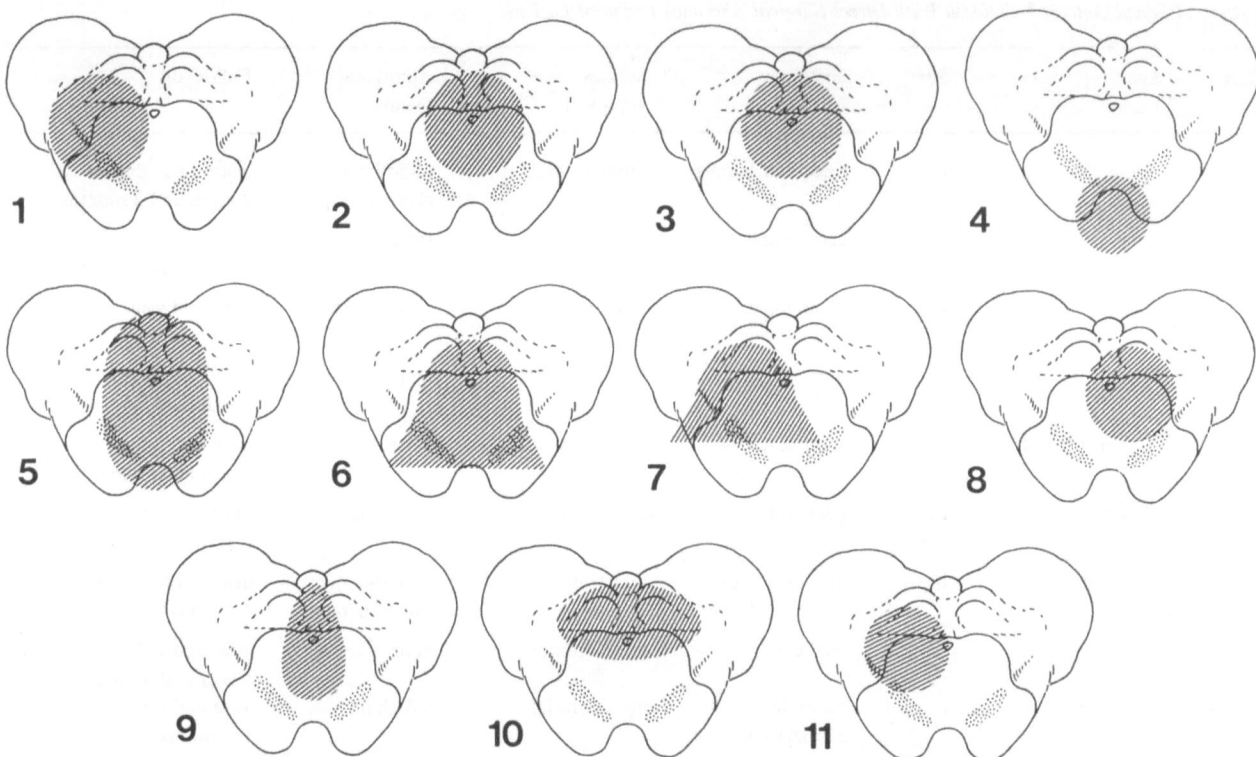

Fig. 1. Schematic presentation of the localisation of 11 surgically approached intrinsic midbrain lesions from Table 2

Table 3. *Clinical Data in 5 Non-Surgical Cases With Lesions of the Pineal-Midbrain Region*

Case no.	Age	Sex	Localization and tentative diagnosis	Signs and symptoms	Causes of conservative management and follow-up
1	6 years	f	calcified lesions, left midbrain	hypesthesia of left facial side, mild spasticity of the right leg since infancy	no indication; follow-up 4 years with improvement of clinical signs
2	8 years	m	cystic lesion in the pineal region	short history of personality change with increased tiredness and polyphagia	no consent by parents, death 1 month after localization, no post mortem
3	7 years	f	small cystic lesion in the pineal region	personality change	improving, no indication, close observation for 2 years
4	10 years	m	cystic lesion of the pineal region, cells in CSF suggested dysgerminoma	progressive personality change, hearing loss	no consent by parents, 2 years follow-up
5	3 years	m	partially, calcified lesion, right midbrain	progressive ataxia	no consent by parents, no follow-up

Table 4. *Histology of 20 Lesions of the Pineal Region in Children 1973–1984*

	Pineal	Midbrain
Pineocytoma	1	
Germinoma	2	
Pilocytic astrocytoma	1	2
Astrocytoma II		1
Astrocytoma III		1
Ependymoma		1
Ependymoblastoma		1
Medulloblastoma	1	2
Glial tumor (open biopsy)		1
Primitive neuroectodermal tumor	1	
Hamartoma		1
Glial cyst	2	
Arachnoid cyst	1	
Hematoma		1
Total	9	11

operatively (case 5 of the midbrain series); this is equivalent to an incidence of operative deaths of 5% among 20 surgical cases. Death due to the primary disease occurred in cases with highly malignant tumors despite radiotherapy and chemotherapy.

Despite dramatic pre-operative courses with severe neurological signs and symptoms all survivors experienced marked improvement, the quality of survival in all cases was good to excellent, except in two of the midbrain series with deficits, which were also markedly improved by surgery (case 4 and case 9).

Discussion

Modern neuroimaging methods help to decide whether to approach a lesion in the deep midline region of the brain and brainstem surgically or confine treatment to CSF diversion and radiotherapy or to close observation.

A histological diagnosis of the lesion is necessary before radiotherapy is administered. For many neurosurgeons stereotactic biopsy for histological diagnosis is still the treatment of choice.

The appropriate therapy, whether radiological or surgical can be now selected on a more rational basis (Conway 1973).

Biological markers, like HCG and AFP, as indicators of germ cell tumors may suggest primary radiotherapy.

In our own series the histology of 20 cases with surgical exposure as listed in Table 4 showed that at least 9 of the lesions were entirely benign and unresponsive either to radiotherapy or chemotherapy.

In another 2 cases, *i.e.,* astrocytoma II and ependymoma, this treatment as a sole alternative to open surgery is questionable.

Whether to attack a pineal region tumor surgically or not is no longer a matter of debate for many authors, since modern microneurosurgical equipment provides a safe approach to radiologically well delineated lesions and optimum post-operative care has become available. But what is the appropriate surgical route has not been settled yet, since surgical methods vary from one centre to the other. We consider the infratentorial supracerebellar approach to be the safest for pineal tumors above the quadrigeminal plate and less mutilating (Stein 1971) than the transcallosal approach (Hoffman 1984) which, although associated with a high mortality in the past but, is still favoured by some. Many authors appreciate the occipital transtentorial approach (Heppner 1959, Poppen 1966); the resection of the occipital pole as published by Horrax (1937) for very large tumors will be confined to very rare cases. Intrinsic lesions of the midbrain, which are not generally considered to be resectable like lesions of the pineal region itself, are only approached by an infratentorial route, mostly in association with additional transection of the cerebellum. Since most of these lesions are clinically similar to those confined to the pineal region itself, the authors group them together as a single entity.

In all of these cases, the decision for surgery should be made on the basis of the same clinical and ethical background as in midline lesions of any other region except the pons and medulla oblongata.

References

1. Conway, L. W., Stereotaxis diagnosis and treatment of intracranial tumors including an initial experience with cryosurgery for pinealomas. J. Neurosurg. *38* (1973), 453–460.
2. Heppner, F., Zur Operationstechnik bei Pinealomen. Zbl. Neurochir. *19* (1959), 219–224.
3. Hoffman, H. J., Transcallosal approach for pineal tumors and the Hospital for Sick Children Series of pineal region tumors. In: Diagnosis and Treatment of Pineal Region Tumors (Neuwelt, E. A., ed.), pp. 223–235. Baltimore-London: Williams and Wilkins. 1984.
4. Horrax, G., Extirpation of a large pinealoma from a patient with pubertas praecox: a new operative approach. Arch. Neurol. Psychiat. *37* (1937), 385–397.
5. Ostertag, C. B., Mennel, H. D., Kiessling, M., Stereotactic biopsy of brain tumors. Surg. Neurol. *14* (1980), 275–283.

6. Pendl, G., Microsurgical anatomy of the pineal region. In: Diagnosis and Treatment of Pineal Region Tumors (Neuwelt, E. A., ed.), pp. 155–207. Baltimore-London: Williams and Wilkins. 1984.
7. Poppen, J. L., The right occipital approach to a pinealoma. J. Neurosurg. *25* (1966), 706–710.
8. Stein, B. M., The infratentorial supracerebellar approach to pineal lesions. J. Neurosurg. *35* (1971), 197–202.

9. Wood, J. H., Zimmerman, R. A., Bruce, D. A., Bilaniuk, L. T., Norris, D. G., Schut, L., Assessment and management of pineal-region and related tumors. Surg. Neurol. *16* (1981), 192–210.

Author's address: Dr. G. Pendl, Associate Professor Neurosurgery, Department of Neurosurgery, University of Vienna Medical School, Währinger Gürtel 18-20, A-1090 Wien, Austria.

Acta Neurochirurgica, Suppl. 35, 119–122 (1985)

Tumors of the Pineal Region in Children and Adolescents

R. Kalff[1], H. E. Clar[1], M. Bamberg[2], and J. Holldack[3]

Departments of Neurosurgery[1], Radiotherapy[2], and Pediatrics[3],
University Essen, Federal Republic of Germany

Summary

The treatment of tumors in the pineal area remains controversial. There are two main approaches:

Conservative treatment, consisting in CSF shunting and radiotherapy, and direct surgical removal.

We report on 25 children (22 boys and 3 girls) aged between 4 and 20 years who underwent conservative treatment. The follow-up period ranges from 1 to 11 years (mean, 4.8 years). 19 patients are still alive at a mean survival time of 5.8 years. 17 children are free of disease, two have severe neurological deficits.

Our diagnostic and therapeutical concepts are presented.

Keywords: Pineal tumor; radiotherapy; CSF shunt; pinealoma.

Introduction

About 3–8% of intracranial tumors in childhood are tumors of the pineal region[1]. Because of their central location and variable morphology (Figure 1, Russel and Rubinstein[7]) their diagnosis and treatment are fraught with problems. Therefore, an individualized management concept is indispensable in these tumors.

Methods and Materials

Our series included 25 children and adolescents (22 boys and 3 girls), aged 4 to 20 years with tumors in the pineal area (Fig. 2). 4 of the patients had ectopic pinealomas; of these, 3 were located in the suprasellar region. In one case a mediastinal mass and a bone lesion had occured two years before the tumor in the pineal area was diagnosed.

The follow-up period was 1 to 11 years (mean, 4.8 years).

Treatment and Results

Because of occlusive hydrocephalus signs of increased intracranial pressure predominated in 20 patients so that CSF shunting was inevitable. Failure of

I germ-cell tumors

  a. germinomas or atypical teratomas
  b. teratoma
  c. teratocarcinoma
  d. choriocarcinoma
  e. endodermal sinus tumor
  f. mixed teratoma and germinoma

II tumors of pineal parenchymal cell origin

  a. pineoblastoma
  b. pinealocytoma

III tumors of other cell origin

  a. gliomas
  b. meningeoma
  c. haemangiopericytoma
  d. melandoma

IV Non-neoplastic cysts and vascular lesions

  a. arachnoid cysts
  b. degenerative cysts
  c. epidermoid cysts
  d. aneurysm of vein of Galen
  e. arteriovenous malformation

Fig. 1. Classification of pineal tumors

upward gaze (Parinaud's Syndrome) was the most common neurological deficit. Patients showed hypothalamic dysfunction in 15 cases. In most of them there was a decrease in somatotropic hormone levels (Fig. 3).

Serum and CSF beta-HCG and AFP levels were elevated in 6 cases.

Tumor cells were present in CSF (Fig. 4) in 11 patients; in 5 cases the tumor cells were identified by cytology (3 pineoblastomas, 1 pinealoma and 1 ependymoma) (Fig. 5).

In 8 of our early cases only the tumor region was irradiated with 50 to 60 Gy.

Children and adolescents with tumor in the pineal region

♂ 22
♀ 3   }   n = 25   mean age 13.1 years

Fig. 2

ENDOCRINOLOGICAL EXAMINATIONS IN CHILDREN WITH PINEAL TUMORS (n =20) HYPOTHALAMIC DYSFUNCTIONS (n=15)

age /sex	somato trop	cortico trop	thyreo trop	gonado trop	diabetes insipidus
5 / ♂	↓				
15 / ♂	↓				
14 / ♂		↓	↓	↓	+
4 / ♂	↓	↓			
16 / ♂	↓	↓			
14 / ♂	↓				
6 / ♂	↓		↓		
15 / ♂	↓	↓	↓	↓	+
12 / ♂					+
15 / ♂	↓	↓		↓	
16 / ♂	↓	↓		↓	+
16 / ♂	↓				
17 / ♂		↓			+
7 / ♀	↓		↓		+
6 / ♂	↓				

Fig. 3

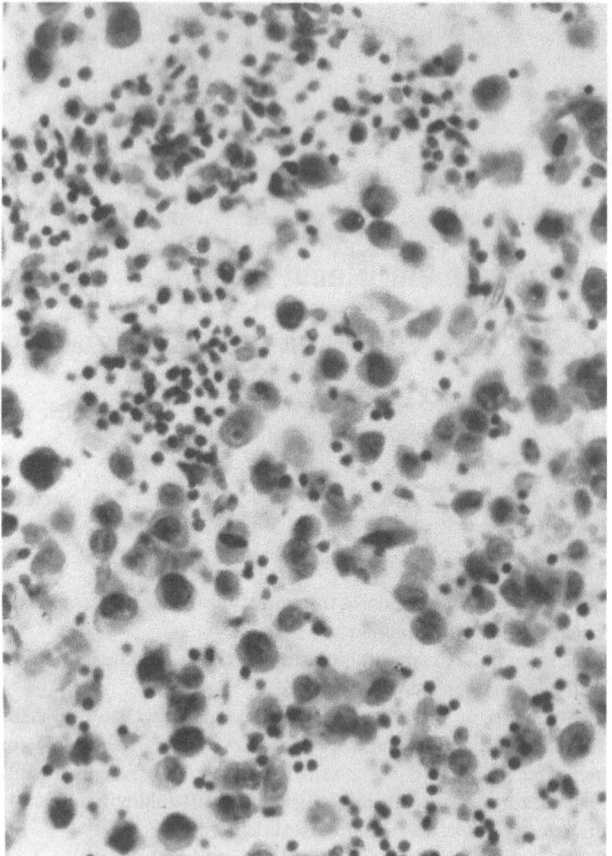

Fig. 4

The following 17 patients received whole brain irradiation with 30 to 40 Gy followed by a boost to the tumor region, the boost dose being 20 to 30 Gy. As tumor cells were present in the CSF in 11 cases, an additional 30 to 38 Gy were rendered to the spinal cord (Fig. 6).

The following case of a 14-year-old boy impressively shows the necessity of whole brain irradiation.

After radiation treatment with a dose of 50 Gy to the pineal region the tumor disappeared (Figs. 7A and B).

18 months later frontal metastasis was seen on CT. Local radiation with 50 Gy was repeated and the tumor again disappeared (Figs. 8A and B). One year later a tumor had developed in the area of the third ventricle. This metastasis can be seen in the space of 1 cm separating the two radiation fields. After local irradiation with 24 Gy no tumor regrowth has been noted yet (Figs. 9A and B).

The boy is well without neurological deficits.

19 patients are still alive at a survival time of 5.8 years. 17 children are free from disease. In 2 cases there are severe neurological deficits caused by increased intracranial pressure because of shunt dysfunction in one case and of epidural hematoma secondary to shunting in the other.

TUMOR CELLS IN CSF
n =11

pinealoblastoma	3
ependymoma	1
pinealoma	1
not identified	6

Fig. 5

RADIATION TREATMENT

tumor region	50 - 60 Gy	8
whole brain and boost to the tumor region	30 - 40 Gy 20 - 30 Gy	6
whole brain and boost to the tumor region and radiation of spinal cord	30 - 38 Gy	11

Fig. 6

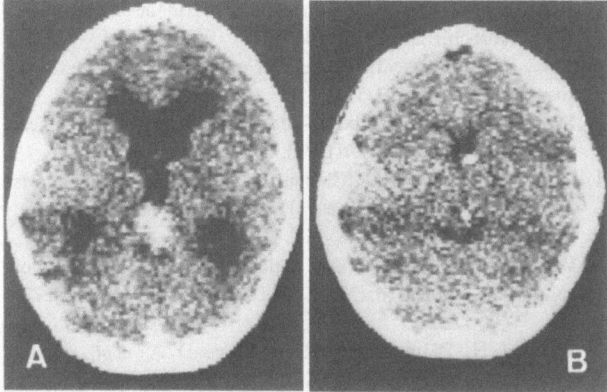

Fig. 7

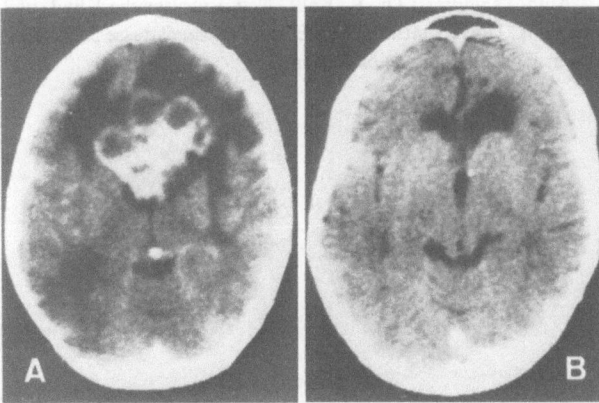

Fig. 8

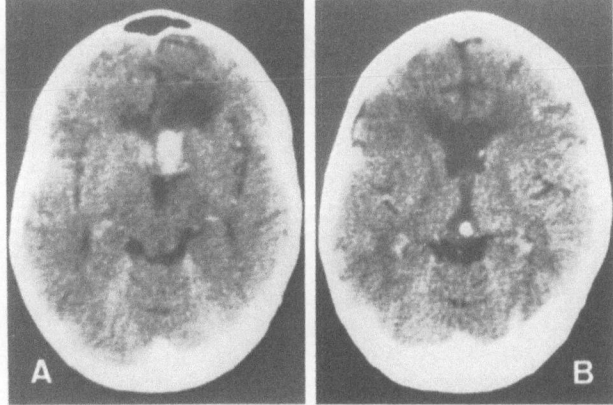

Fig. 9

Endocrinological deficits did not deteriorate after radiotherapy.

There were 6 deaths. One patient died of septicemia and uncontrollable pneumonia. In the remaining 5 progessive tumor growth was the cause of death. This had given rise to spinal metastasis in one case and to a peritoneal secondary in another (Fig. 10).

Alive		19
	diseasefree	17
	severe neurological deficits	2
Dead		6
	progressive growth of tumor	5
	septicemia and pneumonia	1

Fig. 10

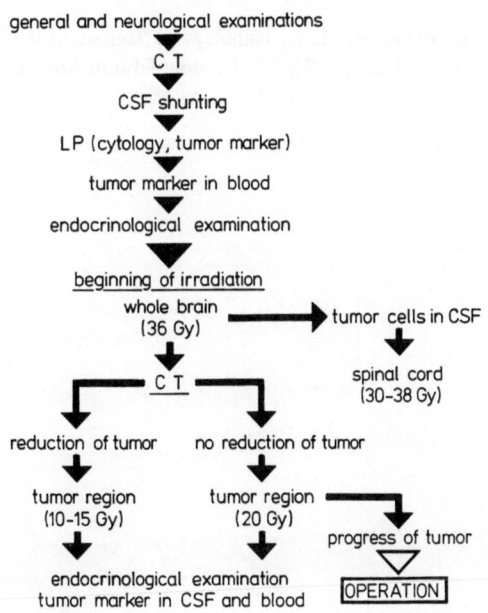

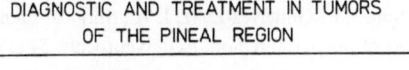

Fig. 11

Discussion

The operating microscope and improvement of microsurgical techniques have given new impetus to attempts at direct surgical removal of tumors in the pineal area. Operative mortality dropped to below 5%[4–6, 8–10, 12, 13]. But long-term follow-up examinations are rare. As about 70% of these tumors are considered to be malignant and ineligible for total removal and because a similar percentage is radiosensitive[2, 3, 11], we are convinced that conservative treatment consisting in CSF shunting and radiotherapy has a place in these cases. If the tumor fails to respond to radiotherapy surgical removal should be attempted.

Encouraged by our results we think that our diagnostic and therapeutic concepts offer a useful approach to the management of tumors in the pineal region (Fig. 11).

References

1. Abay, E. O., Laws, E. R., *et al.*, Pineal tumors in children and adolescents. J. Neurosurg. *55* (1981), 889–895.
2. De Girolami, U., Schmidek, H., Clinico pathological study of 53 tumors of the pineal region. J. Neurosurg. *39* (1973), 455–462.
3. Fowler, F. D., Alexander, E., jr., Davis, C. H., jr., Pinealoma with matastases in the central nervous system. J. Neurosurg. *13* (1956), 271–278.
4. Lazar, M. L., Clark, K., Direct surgical management of masses in the region of the vein of Galen. Surg. Neurol. *2* (1974), 17–21.
5. Neuwelt, E. A., Glasberg, M., Frenkel, E., *et al.*, Malignant pineal region tumors. A clinico-pathological study. J. Neurosurg. *51* (1979), 597–607.
6. Obrador, S., Soto, M., Gutierrez-Diaz, J. A., Surgical management of tumors of the pineal region. Acta Neurochir. *34* (1976), 159–171.
7. Russel, D. S., Rubinstein, L. J., Pathology of Tumors of the Nervous System, 4th ed., pp.283–298. London: Edward Arnold. 1977.
8. Sano, K., Diagnosis and treatment of tumors in the pineal region. Acta Neurochir. *34* (1976), 153–157.
9. Stein, B. M., Surgical treatment of pineal tumors. Clin. Neurosurg. *26* (1979), 490–510.
10. Stein, B. M., Supra cerebellar-infratentorial approach to pineal tumors. Surg. Neurol. *11* (1979), 331–337.
11. Sung, D., Harisiadis, L., Chang, C. H., Midline pineal tumors and suprasellar germinomas: Highly curable by irradiation. Radiology *128* (1978), 745–751.
12. Ventureyra, E. C. G., Pineal region: surgical management of tumors and vascular malformations. Surg.Neurol. *16* (1981), 77–84.
13. Wood, J. H., Zimmermann, R. A., Bruce, D. A., *et al.*, Assessment and management of pineal-region and related tumors. Surg. Neurol. *16* (1981).

Author's address: Dr. R. Kalff, Neurochirurgische Klinik und Poliklinik, Universitätsklinikum Essen, Hufelandstrasse 55, D-4300 Essen, Federal Republic of Germany.

Acta Neurochirurgica, Suppl. 35, 123–125 (1985)

I. Brain Stem

Direct Surgical Attack on Pontine and Rhombencephalic Lesions

F. Heppner, R. W. Oberbauer, and **P. W. Ascher**

Neurosurgical Department, University of Graz, Austria

Summary

The introduction of lasers in neurosurgery in 1976 can be considered as a major contribution to gaining access to "untouchable" areas of the brain. This immaterial instrument provides for precise cutting at low penetration depth in surrounding tissues and may carbonize, and thus remove, layers not to be touched because of their highly sensitive vicinity.

From a total of 794 patients experiencing the advantages of laser surgery (1976–1984), a series of 12 children with lower brainstem tumors is presented. Intraoperative instability of vital functions was absent throughout, leaving the patients without deterioriation of their initial neurological condition. Given appropriate handling and adequate experience, the laser is a singularly helpful surgical tool for gaining access to areas hitherto barred to surgery.

Keywords: Laser surgery, lower brainstem, pediatric age.

Introduction

After intensive experimental investigations of the effects of different lasers on nervous tissue[1, 2, 15], the CO_2 laser (type Sharplan 791) was introduced in neurosurgery by Heppner and Ascher in 1976[1, 6–8]. This immaterial instrument turned out to be singularly helpful in lesions which either originated in or were closely related to structures of the midline. These deserve special attention because, while often actually being malignant, they had to be considered "malignant" due to their localization, even if benign. Prior to the use of lasers, the vast majority of lower brainstem lesions had to be treated conservatively, as mechanical or electrical dissection was incompatible with basic vital functions. Using the CO_2 laser, lesions in the pons and medulla oblongata have, however, been shown to be amenable to surgery without interference with respiration, pulse rate and blood pressure.

The advantages of the CO_2 laser, which the authors had occasion to appreciate in a total of 794 procedures, are as follows:

1. The focused laser beam cuts precisely and with low penetration depth. Accordingly, the cut surfaces are sharp and smooth.

2. By increasing the distance of the handpiece from the surface, the defocused beam produces an enhanced heat effect on nervous tissue, which can be used for coagulation and carbonisation of tumor residues. Consequently, these can be removed in layers by microsuction until normal brain tissue is reached.

3. The laser beam can be combined with the operating microscope and thus offers optimal precision by focused application. Technical data of different lasers have been published elsewhere[1, 3, 6, 9].

Material and Results

From 1950–1984 a total of 347 pediatric patients (age, 0–15 years) underwent surgery for brain tumors. Of these, 168 were located supratentorially and a slight majority of 179 were infratentorial. This is in agreement with other larger series[12, 14]. Out of the total of 162 patients with midline lesions, 12 with tumors of the lower brainstem, i.e. pons and medulla oblongata, were operated with the CO_2 laser. The essential features of this subgroup (localization, histology and type of laser application) are listed in Table 1. We had three deaths of which only one was directly related to the operative procedure. The remaining 9 patients of this series survived without neurological deterioration. It should be stressed that intraoperative instability of vital functions was absent throughout.

Figure 1 shows the CT scan of a pontine lesion compressing the fourth ventricle. The surface of the pons apparently bulges into the operating field (Fig. 2). After splitting the pons (Fig. 3), gross resection of the well demarcated mass was accomplished bringing into view the arachnoid of the pontine cistern (Fig. 4). The patient, a boy of 3 years fully, recovered 4 weeks after the procedure.

Table 1. *Essential Data of This Series (lower brain stem tumors, n = 12)*

Type of tumor	Number	Location	Type of surgery	Type of laser application	Operative mortality
Medulloblastoma	2	rhomboid fossa	2 resection	preparation and vaporation	0
	1	pons	1 resection	preparation	
Glioblastoma	1	pons	1 probatoria	preparation	0
Astrocytoma	2	rhomboid fossa	2 exstirpation	preparation and vaporation	1 pulmonary embolism
	2	pons	1 biopsy 1 resection	preparation	1 edema
Spongioblastoma	2	pons rhomboid fossa	1 biopsy 1 extirpation	preparation preparation	0 intestinnal hemorrhage
Ependymoma	2	rhomboid fossa	2 resection	preparation and vaporation	0

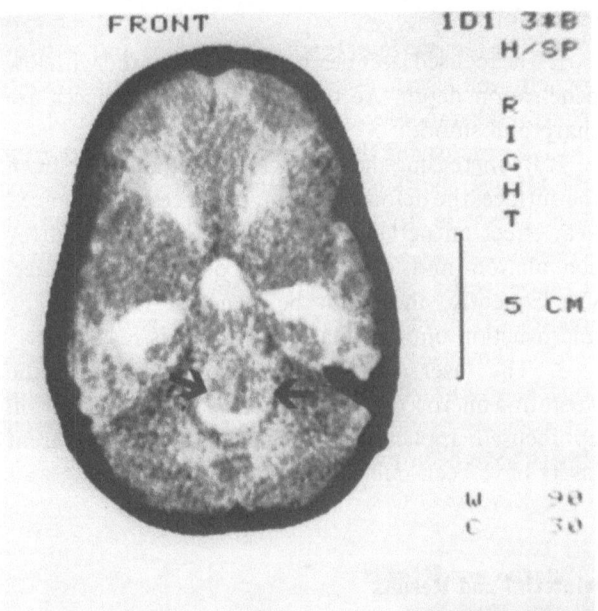

Fig. 1. CT-Scan: Isodense lesion of the pons (arrows) compressing the fourth ventricle

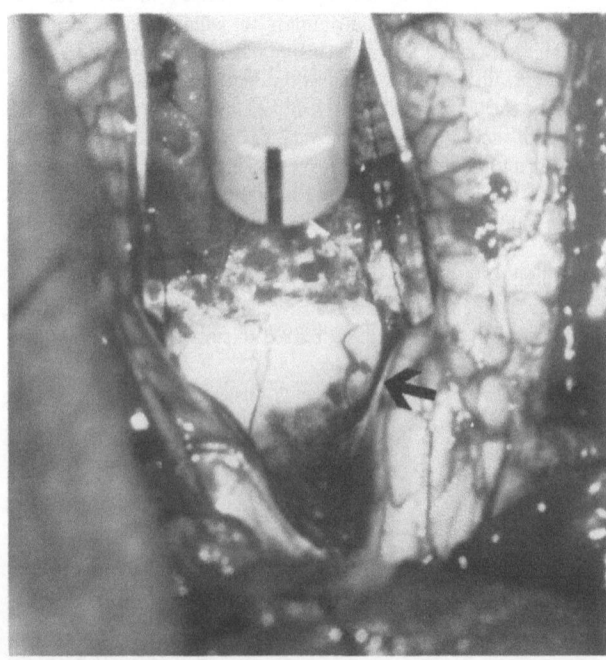

Fig. 2. Laser handpiece pointing at the pontine area in the fourth ventricle (arrow), apparently bulging into the operating field

Discussion

Surgery of tumors in the lower brainstem has been and will continue to be considered one of the most delicate procedures in neurosurgery. Reports in the literature suggested these tumors to be inoperable until a few years ago, when reports about successfull operative treatment have been published[1, 6, 11, 16, 22]. The tremendous technical advances of recent years have provided an even more sophisticated approach to such locations so that tumor removal may be accomplished with satisfactory results[4-6, 10-12, 18, 21]. Although the present series comprises a very limited number of cases, one fact established in a far larger number of adult patients also holds true for children: Using a special operative technique, surgery of the lower brainstem can be survived without any additional damage and can thus be definitely helpful. However, a clear distinction must be made between well demarcated neoplasms and diffusely growing tumors of the lower brainstem, which remain inoperable.

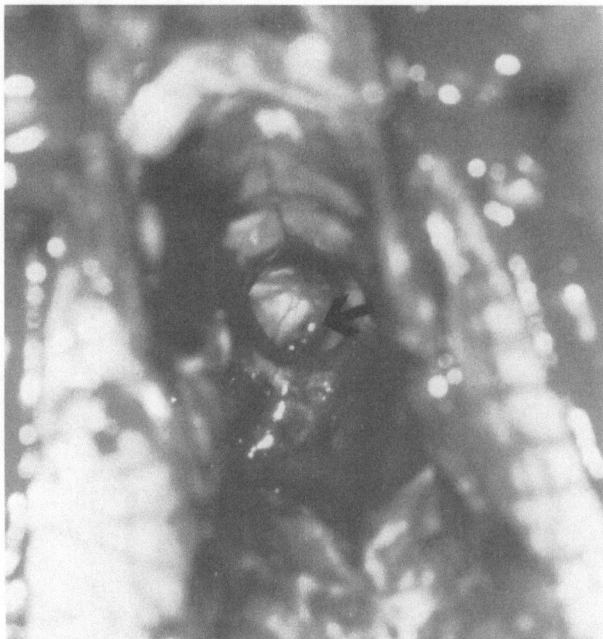

Fig. 3. Pontine incision (arrow) after partial tumor removal

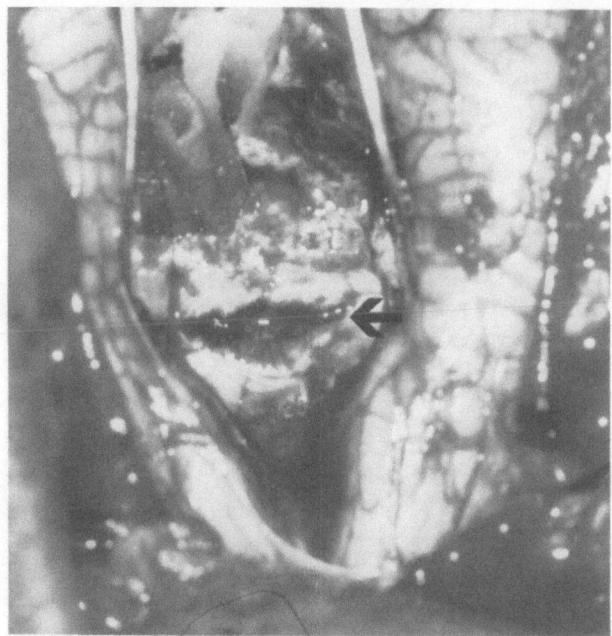

Fig. 4. Same view after tumor removal. Arrow points at the arachnoid of the pontine cistern

References

1. Alvisi, C., Cerisoli, M., Maccheroni, M. E., Long-term results of surgically treated brainstem gliomas. Acta Neurochir. (Wien) *76*, 12–17.
2. Ascher, P. W., Der CO_2-Laser in der Neurochirurgie. Wien: Molden. 1977.
3. Ascher, P. W., Oberbauer, R. W., Ingolitsch, E., Walter, G., Neuere histologische Untersuchungsergebnisse nach Gebrauch des Lasers am Zentralnervensystem, Kongressber. *19*. Tagung d. Öst. Ges. f. Chir., pp. 479–483. Wien: H. Egermann. 1978.
4. Ascher, P. W., Cerullo, L., Chapter 9: Laser Use in Neurosurgery. In: Surgical Applications of Lasers, pp. 163–174. Chicago: Year Book Medical Publ. 1983.
5. Ascher, P. W., Absolute inoperable tumors have to be reconsidered under the use of different lasers. Third Congress on Laser Neurosurgery (1984) Summaries, p. 192. Chicago, May 7–9, 1984.
6. Entzian, W., Removal of low brain stem spongioblastomas—positive long term results in circumscribed lesions. Proc. 12th Scientific Meeting, Int. Society for Pediatric Neurosurgery, Cairo, Sept. 1984.
7. Heppner, F., Ascher, P. W., Über den Einsatz des Laserstrahls in der Neurochirurgie. Medizinalmarkt *12* (1976), 424–426.
8. Heppner, F. Ascher, P. W., Hirnoperationen mit dem CO_2-Laser. Melsunger Med. Mitt. *51*, Suppl. II (1977), 121–123.
9. Heppner, F., Ascher, P. W., The use of laser in neurosurgery. 6th Int. Congr. of Neurol. Surgery, Abstr. *418*, (Excerpta Med. Publ.), p. 134. Sao Paulo, Jun. 19–25, 1977.
10. Heppner, F., Ascher, P. W., Operationen an Hirn und Rückenmark mit dem CO_2-Laser. Acta Chir. Austriaca *9* (1977), 32–34.
11. Heppner, F., Ascher, P. W., Oberbauer, R. W., Surgery of brain stem tumours in children. Acta Neurochir. (Wien) *62* (1982).
12. Hoffmann H. J., Becker, L., Craven, M. A., A clinically and pathologically distinct group of benign brain stem gliomas. Neurosurgery *7* (1980), 243–248.
13. Hooper, R., Intracranial tumors in childhood. Childs Brain *1* (1975), 136–140.
14. Ingraham, F. D., Matson, D. D., Neurosurgery of Infancy and Childhood. Springfield, Ill., U.S.A.: Ch. C Thomas. 1954.
15. Koos W. T., Miller, M. H., Intracranial Tumors of Infants and Children. Stuttgart: Thieme. 1971.
16. Lassiter, K. R. L., Alexander, E., Courtland, D., Jr., David, L. K., Jr.: Surgical treatment of brain-stem gliomas. J. Neurosurg. *34* (1971), 719–724.
17. Oberbauer, R. W., Ascher, P. W., Ingolitsch, E., Walter, C., Ultrastructural findings in CNS tissue with CO_2-laser. Congr. Rep. Laser Surgery Vol. II, pp. 81–90. Jerusalem: Academic Press. 1978.
18. Oberbauer, R. W., Heppner, F., Ascher, P. W., Surgery of tumors in the midline. Proc. 8th Meeting European Society for Pediatric Neurosurgery, Rennes, Jun. 27–30, 1982, p. 24.
19. Olivecroma, H., The surgical treatment of intracranial tumors. In: Handbuch der Neurochirurgie 4/IV, p. 99. Berlin-Heidelberg-New York: Springer. 1967.
20. Panitch, H. S., Berg, B. O., Brain stem tumors of childhood and adolescence. Am. J. Dis. Child *119* (1970), 465–472.
21. Reigel, D. H., Brain-Stem Tumors During Childhood. In: Pediatric Neurosurgery. Grune and Stratton. 1982.
22. Strange, P., Wohlert, L.: Primary brain stem tumours. Acta Neurochir. (Wien) *62* (1982), 219–232.
23. Tönnis, W., Diagnostik der intrakraniellen Geschwülste. In: Handbuch der Neurochirurgie 4/III, pp. 308–309. Berlin-Göttingen-Heidelberg: Springer. 1962.

Authors' address: O. Univ.-Prof. Dr. F. Heppner, OA. Dr. Rainer Oberbauer, Univ. Prof. Dr. Peter Wolf Ascher, Universitäts-Klinik für Neurochirurgie, Landeskrankenhaus, A-8036 Graz, Austria.